RESTORING
YOUR EYESIGHT

RESTORING
YOUR EYESIGHT

A TAOIST APPROACH

DOUG MARSH

FOREWORD BY
THOMAS R. QUACKENBUSH

Healing Arts Press
Rochester, Vermont

Healing Arts Press
One Park Street
Rochester, Vermont 05767
HealingArtsPress.com

Healing Arts Press is a division of Inner Traditions International

Note to the Reader: *This book is intended as an informational guide. The remedies,
approaches, and techniques described herein are meant to supplement, and not to
be a substitute for, professional medical care or treatment. They should not be used
to treat a serious ailment without prior consultation with a qualified health care
professional.*

LIBRARY OF CONGRESS CATALOGING-IN-PUBLICATION DATA
Marsh, Doug.
    Restoring your eyesight : a Taoist approach / Doug Marsh ; foreword by
Thomas R. Quackenbush.
        p. cm.
    Summary: "A holistic guide to improving one's vision both physically and
spiritually"—Provided by publisher.
    ISBN-13: 978-1-59477-150-7
    ISBN-10: 1-59477-150-2
    1. Vision disorders—Alternative treatment. 2. Visual training. 3. Taoism.
I. Title.
    RE48.M39 2007
    617.7—dc22
                                                                    2006026086

Printed and bound in the United States by Lake Book Manufacturing

10   9   8   7   6   5   4   3   2   1

Text design and layout by Rachel Goldenberg
This book was typeset in Sabon and Avenir with Copperplate and Avenir as the
display typefaces

To send correspondence to the author of this book, mail a first-class letter to the
author c/o Inner Traditions • Bear & Company, One Park Street, Rochester, VT
05767, and we will forward the communication.

CONTENTS

FOREWORD

In May 1999 I received a lengthy e-mail from Doug Marsh regarding his interest in Natural Vision Improvement (NVI). Over the last seven years we have had many communications on this topic.

Now Doug contributes *Restoring Your Eyesight: A Taoist Approach* to the relatively sparse and much needed library of NVI books in his "motivation to reach out to others." I am surprised and pleased to discover Doug's book is on par (yes, a pun on his love of golf!) with books written by professional NVI teachers.

His theme of Taoism is appropriate, since both NVI and Taoism teach a way of life that is in balance and harmony with nature—something many of us have not yet achieved, not by conscious choice, but because of the severe imbalances that modern culture presents to us. Taoist philosophy includes "rhythm, softness, return, balance, and wholeness." There has hardly been a better description of the attributes associated with good eyesight. In my work, I use the right brain/left brain theme, which ultimately steers us toward the same goal of good eyesight. Both philosophies emphasize relaxation, movement, and centralization (which Doug has coined "concentric focus"). These principles are presented and described very well herein.

The damage caused by modern industrialization and technology is explored in part 1, "Excess." Why are the majority of people living in "civilized" societies unable to function normally—without crutches on their noses or in their eyes? Doug presents good answers.

The ancient wisdom of Taoism as related to NVI fundamentals are primarily offered in part 2, "The Way." It is important to understand that NVI really is "a way." Most students of NVI understand it to be a series of eye exercises done for twenty minutes per day. However, this is not entirely correct. NVI is a process of relearning how to see the correct way—the way most of us learn naturally, automatically, and subconsciously in the first year of our lives. Dr. Bates stated that these are "habits" and are meant to be used "all day long." And as I like to remind my students, anyone can relearn something they used to do perfectly.

I should add that a specific spiritual teaching is not needed to improve one's eyesight, however, the philosophical concepts common to both *are* needed. On an amusing note, I once had a potential student tell me she did not want to attend my classes after attending a free introductory lecture, because she concluded I was teaching "Presbyterian" vision. Just for the record, I had only discussed "presbyopic" vision, no religion!

Have you ever seen your vision fluctuate? Perhaps while on vacation you have noticed that you often see better. Or, conversely, when under excessive stress, you may have noticed that your vision is not entirely clear, or even that it is crossed-eyed. Have you ever noticed that after wearing glasses for a few hours and then taking them off, your vision is more blurred than before you put them on? Then, after a few more hours of not wearing them, your vision gets better again? If so, then you have *experienced* NVI, and you have contradicted the theories of virtually all eye doctors who dogmatically proclaim that it is impossible for eyesight to improve naturally. The theory (a guess) that eyesight cannot improve is so ingrained in the orthodox professionals that, sometimes, when improvement is measured and verified, they will say their previous examinations were in error! That may not be a reassuring thought to many people!!

An optician once told one of my students that she (the optician) only needed her stronger glasses when she was under high stress. Since vision fluctuates for everyone, and most people know this, it is curious that eye professionals, in their professional practice, adhere so strongly to theories that contradict their own experience. As a holistic dentist once stated, "They can't teach you what they don't know; and they can't lead you were they won't go." Go to authorities who have been taught that your eyesight cannot get better naturally and have no experience with people's eyesight improving naturally, and most likely you will not improve. Go to authorities who have been taught eyesight *can* improve naturally and have lots of experience with people's eyesight improving, and your chances are a lot better. Flaws and confusion within the optometric and ophthalmologic professions are covered in part 3, "Harmony."

Doug's writings include his own struggles with glasses and contact lenses, as he wonders how, for instance, to rid himself of these torturous crutches—an all too common plight of people all over the world. The theories of myopia being hereditary, and presbyopia being due to old age, are shattered by simple facts. But to what *can* we attribute myopia and presbyopia? Dr. Bates showed us that they are due to stress—not just any stress, but specific strained, mental, emotional, and physical vision habits. In a wonderful way, Doug helps us to understand terms like "force, stress, strain, pressure, and tension," and "concentration"—terms that are often misunderstood. By relearning natural vision habits and principles Doug has been rewarded with excellent improvement "accumulated dramatically over the long run"—as have I. Thomas Chavez, a homeopath and one of my NVI students, in his book *Body Electronics,* defines health as freedom, which resonates with Doug's own NVI process as being "a liberating journey."

Doug describes many supportive holistic therapies including massage, Feldenkrais, Alexander Technique, craniosacral therapy, and myofascial release. Any therapy that truly supports relaxation, movement (circulation), and centralization (relaxed visual concentration) will accelerate the improvement of one's eyesight.

Since there is a strong correlation between certain "functional" vision problems (nearsightedness, farsightedness, and presbyopia for example) and eye disease, many people are also seeking NVI for preventative reasons. Ignorance is not bliss when it comes to eyesight.

Bottom line? Lower the power of your prescription glasses and/or contact lenses (safely and legally if for driving), use your own eyes more and more, and restore your eyesight by relearning natural vision habits and principles. Since 1983 I have watched thousands of my own students improve their vision. Many thousands more have improved under the tutelage of other NVI teachers. Educate yourself and reap the rewards!

I believe Doug's book will be a valuable aid for those seeking the truth about eyesight and how to take care of it in a natural way. In fact, I will now be using Doug's excellent information in my NVI classes. Motivation, patience, perseverance, and commitment are necessary, but the rewards are—most likely—far beyond what one might currently expect.

As one reader of my book stated, this process "could actually be called *Relearning to Live*."

Sounds Taoist to me.

THOMAS R. QUACKENBUSH

Thomas R. Quackenbush is a vision educator whose seminal book *Relearning to See* fully articulates the Bates Method of natural vision improvement.

Introduction

A tree as great as a man's embrace springs from a small
  shoot;
A terrace nine stories high begins with a pile of earth;
A journey of a thousand miles starts under one's feet.

The bright path seems dim;
Going forward seems like retreat;
The easy way seems hard.

Lao Tzu[1]

THE SEED

Without warning, my blurry vision spontaneously cleared to virtually 20/20 sight for a few seconds. At that moment I knew what the expression "breathtaking" meant; the sheer exhilaration almost caused me to stop breathing. My stunned reaction occurred because my high-prescription "Coke-bottle" glasses were in my coat pocket while I was walking along the sidewalk! It had been almost thirty-five years since I'd been able to see that clearly and naturally with my own eyes, unaided by the artificial clarity of strong glasses.

I'd heard of people having a religious experience or a spiritual awakening. Whether the emotional surge I had at that moment of sudden visual clarity could be described in such potentially life-altering terms, I can't say for sure. Regardless of the significance of such an overpowering sensation, the event dramatically changed my notions about eyesight and vision health. It gave me a whole new "outlook" on life.

The reason my glasses were in my pocket that day wasn't because I'd broken them. Rather, I had been purposely not wearing them for long periods as part of my experiment with Natural Vision Improvement (NVI), also called the Bates Method. A few weeks earlier, I had purchased an obscure paperback originally published in 1929 entitled *Better Eyesight Without Glasses,* by Harry Benjamin. I had been following Benjamin's advice each day when, out of the blue, I was rewarded with such remarkable yet fleeting clarity. The planted seed had begun to germinate.

Not only has my commitment to improving my eyesight by natural means been personally fulfilling, it has also been a motivation to reach out to others. My NVI "tree" has branched out to bear fruit in the form of the book you are reading.

TAO

You may once have said to someone, "The journey of a thousand miles begins with a single step" and not realized you were dispensing a gem of Taoist wisdom. If you're unfamiliar with Taoism, its origins date back about twenty-five hundred years ago to a wise old man by the name of Lao Tzu (other variations: Lao Tse or Laozi). Legend has it that this mysterious man wrote the Tao Te Ching (pronounced "dow deh jing"). The immense wisdom contained in this surprisingly short but classic work is truly remarkable. Good things do come in small packages, because the Tao Te Ching is a lucid masterpiece on the art of living. The messages are both philosophical and spiritual. Learning to be guided by the inner rather than the outer light is a huge part of coming to grips with what life throws us. Understanding the concept of *inner* and *outer* vision is equally relevant in regaining the purity and clarity of natural eyesight.

The theme on which this book is based is the concept of *Tao*. It is an elusive term that is difficult to precisely translate into English. The first parallel that Westerners may immediately think of is God, but the Tao is not defined as a personal, judgmental deity. According to Huston Smith, it is literally translated as "Way" or "Path"; it's the mystical way of reality, the eternal rhythm in the universe, nature, and human life.[2] George Lucas's *Star Wars* characters could perhaps just as easily have said, "May the Tao be with you." Or instead of "going with the flow," we could say we're "going with the Tao."

Tao Te Ching, then, can be roughly translated as "The Book of the Way" or "The Way and Its Power." The over forty different English versions of the ancient Chinese text give an indication of just how challenging is the task of creating a definitive translation. The versions I've chosen to quote throughout the book are by Gia-fu Feng and Jane English, Thomas Cleary, Ellen M. Chen, and Stephen Mitchell.

JOURNEY

My introduction to the world of prescription eyewear began in grade four. As I sat in the classroom one day, the desk suddenly seemed to move around me. The entire room then started to spin. The vertigo attack left me queasy and clammy, and I obviously didn't look well to the teacher. The next thing I recall was visiting the school nurse's office, where my vision was tested by having me read an eye chart. The nurse recommended an eye examination by a specialist. Whether it was an optometrist or an ophthalmologist, I don't know, but the result was my first pair of glasses.

The novelty of wearing glasses was fun at the beginning. But the novelty quickly wore off; the fun turned to loathing as my lenses got thicker each year. The impediment of glasses led me to reflect about my fate more than once: Why do I have such lousy eyesight? If people in ancient times had vision this poor, how did they function before glasses were invented? How on earth did they manage to do things and get around with such blurry sight?

I also remember reading that my condition, myopia (also called nearsightedness), was hereditary. This made absolutely no sense to me at the time. Neither of my two brothers was nearsighted. Nor did my parents have myopia as children (although they did eventually get glasses as adults, their prescriptions were very weak compared to mine). None of my grandparents had glasses for myopia when they were young either. My instincts were giving me a message that something was amiss.

As an adult, I eventually converted to contact lenses for a more natural appearance, but I soon found as many irritating (literally!) things to despise about them as with glasses. Then one day while I was reading an alternative health magazine dedicated to nutrition and good lifestyle habits, I came across a very brief reference to a controversial eye doctor by the name of William Horatio Bates. The piece stated he had written a book in the early 1900s entitled *The Cure for Imperfect Sight by Treatment Without Glasses*. I immediately "knew" my childhood instincts were right. I was convinced from the start that this was another example of suppression by conventional medicine, the same establishment that once supported tobacco use, claiming it was harmless to health. Although I was unable to locate a copy of Bates's rare book, I did find Harry Benjamin's book, loosely based on Bates's original work. This was my first step on the journey of NVI.

Benjamin suffered from severe myopia at a very early age. He was only four years old when he was prescribed very strong lenses. His eyesight progressively worsened in his youth until age twenty-six, when he was prescribed the strongest lenses the opticians could offer. The eye doctor advised him to quit reading, since the strain could very well endanger his eyes, resulting in more serious problems and even permanent blindness. Benjamin was saved from this grim prognosis when a friend gave him a copy of Bates's book. Because Benjamin was not supposed to read, his brother read the book aloud to him. It was over a year after he began practicing the method in earnest that Benjamin could read his first book without glasses, "very slowly and painfully." At the time his book was published, he said, "It is now two-and-a-half years since I left off my glasses, and I am able to read and write quite well. My distance vision is not so good, but I see sufficiently well to be able to get about all over the place with ease and comfort."[3]

Reading about Benjamin's personal improvement was both inspirational and cautionary. This method was obviously no miracle or instant remedy, yet it did seem to have some merit. Although my nearsightedness was considered high myopia, it was nowhere near the severity of his extreme myopia. If he could benefit as he did, surely the method would help me improve my vision. I had no idea how long it would take or what was in store, but I was motivated to get started and saw no risk in trying. Nothing ventured, nothing gained.

The path was indeed dim, because there was no orthodox support locally. There were also no Bates instructors nearby (at the time I didn't even know people taught his method), so all I had to guide me was Benjamin's information. I soon had the unexpected and surprising glimpse of near-perfect vision that I previously described. That brief period of clarity confirmed that the method was working.

At that stage, I was hopeful my rate of improvement would be fairly swift, yet it wasn't to be. The path of improvement was a long journey that seemed to retreat many times. It also felt slow, lonely, and frustrating, and I considered giving up more than once. But I remembered Benjamin's advice to have "faith, patience, and determination." Taoism also reminded me to be patient: "He who strides cannot maintain the pace."[4]

I yearned to get my hands on Bates's writings to find out what I might be missing or perhaps doing wrong. Eventually the Internet arrived, and this opened up a wealth of information about the Bates Method. I studied several books on NVI, including a reprint of Bates's original 1920 book. These books explained many of the phenomena I had been experiencing on my own. The material helped solidify my belief that NVI was the proper path to follow. My vision has continually improved because of my conviction to stay the course. The gains have been gradual, but they've accumulated dramatically over the long run.

For example, early in my NVI program I took the plunge with naked eyes during office meetings to help wean myself from the strong prescription lenses. My natural sight at that point was so fuzzy (technically, I was legally blind without glasses) that I had tremendous difficulty making out facial features of people three feet across the table from me. The eyes, nose, and mouth of a person's face would be awash in a homogenous, skin-toned hue. My vision gradually improved—month by month, year by year—beyond this abysmal state to a point where I could see remarkably well at much greater distances, even under low light conditions.

I eventually got to the point where I could function quite well without the aid of prescription eyewear for most activities, including golfing. It was during a golf game with my wife late one summer evening that I realized how far I'd come since I started the journey. We were getting in the last couple of holes at dusk, and I was relying solely on my natural eyesight. While standing on the teebox of a par-four 396 yards long, I looked toward the green and could see the flag on the pin distinctly from that distance. I also watched the player ahead, carrying his golf bag on his shoulder, walking on the front fringe of the green.

I mentioned my observations to my wife without a response (she'd gotten so used to my reports of improved clarity that she had became blasé). So when I mentioned it again, she decided to test me. She asked what color the flag was. There were three possible choices depending on where the hole was cut—blue for back of green, yellow for the middle, or red for the front. Without hesitation, I answered yellow, because that's clearly what I saw—no guessing. Although she verified it, the confirmation wasn't necessary; I *knew* what I had seen was correct.

At the risk of sounding melodramatic, I can assure you that the before-and-after states feel remarkably different. Sure there was clarity with artificial lenses, but the vision was very harsh, distorted, and two-dimensional. The world was also a very frightening and threatening place; the strain and adaptation required to see through powerful, rigid glasses under constantly varying lighting conditions throughout each day took a real physical and psychological toll. With good vision the way nature intended, the world is a sight to behold! I marvel at the true depth perception, shimmering colors, and vivid textures. I actually have the sensation that I'm fully immersed in my surroundings, not just a spectator. My natural vision at its clearest moments brings about a relaxed, euphoric, and blissful state of body and mind that I never before knew was possible. Stumbling upon the road of vision improvement has been a blessing and a multifaceted adventure. Most of all, it's been a liberating journey.

THE WAY FROM EXCESS

This book is divided into three sections. Part 1, "Excess," explores the harmful effect of industrialization and technology on the vision health of the populace. Experts have been studying the eye from many different angles for over a couple of centuries, yet the researchers seem no closer to understanding how vision really works than when the quest first started. Several theories suggest how the eye "probably" focuses, and at least nineteen theories have been postulated about the cause of myopia.[5]

Opinions also vary widely on how to treat myopia. Many vision professionals firmly believe that myopia is neither preventable nor reversible, a belief that conforms to the orthodox view in Bates's day. Others believe the condition is preventable but irreversible, while precious few believe it to be both preventable and reversible. All this muddled science would be whimsical if the consequences weren't so dire. Myopic children not only become addicted to prescription lenses for a lifetime of dependence, but their vision continues to deteriorate because of this dependency. Studies indicate that myopia is a major factor behind vision impairment and blindness in adults.[6]

It was within this depressing framework that Bates abandoned orthodox theories and methods of treatment. Part 2 of this book, "The Way," leads you away from the excesses of technology by meshing the ancient wisdom and values of Taoist philosophy—rhythm, softness, return, balance, and wholeness—with the important principles of Bates's teachings.

This section is intended to guide you onto the path of improved vision (and, as a bonus, improved general health). The crux of NVI can best be summed up by the message I found in a fortune cookie one night at a local Chinese restaurant: "Nature, time, and patience are the three great physicians."

The final section, part 3, "Harmony," tackles the flaws in a scientific and educational system that can create such fragmentation within vision science and cause such negativity and suppression of alternatives. It calls for a united front in vision care.

PART ONE

EXCESS

*The Way of heaven
reduces excess and fills need,
but the way of humans is not so.*

LAO TZU

1
THE CHASE

Colors blind people's eyes,
sounds deafen their ears;
flavors spoil people's palates,
the chase and the hunt
craze people's minds.

LAO TZU[1]

Spring is an especially welcome season in Canada, marking the renewal phase after a long winter. That's why gardening is very popular; people are eager to begin their annual green-thumbed rituals. They sow seeds in neat rows and then anxiously wait for the first sprouts to pop through the soil. They continue to nurture and tend their gardens to reap the succulent fruits of their labors. Patience and care are needed, for the gardeners would never think to interfere with nature's miracle of plant life.

Ellen Chen relates the "tragic consequences of human intervention" in the story of a farmer who was concerned his rice plants were not growing quickly enough. When he returned home one day, he told his family, "I am worn out . . . I have been helping the rice plants grow." His wife, realizing what her husband had done, rushed out to the field only to find the plants all shriveled up. He'd been pulling on the plants to help them grow faster.[2]

Western civilization is "modeled on animal life and characterized by struggle, conquest, and the survival of the fittest," says Chen.[3] The excessive use of technological force in the name of progress is exacting a price on our ecology and our society. Are we losing as much as we are gaining in overall health?

RAT RACE

Progress. Industrialization. Machines. Technology. Imagine how intoxicating it was two or three centuries ago to those on the frontier of the changes to come in society. The possibilities must have seemed endless; they dreamed humans would conquer and control the earth and create a mechanistic utopia—heaven on earth—with no disease, no poverty, no famine, no wars.

Most of us living today in Western-style society were raised among machines and systems. There's virtually no escaping them; the few who try are considered Luddites and romantic freaks. The notions of evolution and progress are drilled into us almost from the time we learn to walk and talk. Once fully indoctrinated, many eventually become disillusioned with progress and accept the routine of progress as a rat race. Thomas Cleary explains the opening Lao Tzu quote:

> Colors, sounds, and flavors all have legitimate functions in art, music, and diet, but they are perverted into superficial sensuous diversions. The chase and the hunt represent livelihood from the point of view of effort and struggle, which originally have a function in human life but become diverted into ambition. . . . Livelihood becomes a rat race. People degenerate under these conditions: no longer do they use the energies of sense and feeling to propel themselves into greater understanding and attunement with subtler phenomena such as principles, balances, and harmonies; on the contrary, degenerating humans diffuse energies through the habit of dwelling on the senses and feelings themselves.[4]

Time is money, we're told. With our Western concept of linear time as a fixed commodity, there just doesn't seem to be enough to go around. The hurried, dog-eat-dog pace is given as necessary to get ahead in the world. We have to compete not just with the clock but also with everyone else. Building a better mousetrap is the American dream of rags to riches. Fame and fortune will reward all who work hard enough to achieve it.

Bates had noted in his day, "The various forms of artificial lighting . . . tempt most of us to prolong our vocations and avocations into hours when primitive man was forced to rest."[5] But it's no longer a matter of choice or temptation; industrial society expects and demands that people dutifully push themselves to the limit to succeed. The aberration of punching the clock in mechanical synchronicity has evolved into tossing it aside completely; "nine-to-five" has morphed into "twenty-four/seven," obliterating traditional lines between work and rest. Transcontinental airline pilots, whose schedules drastically flip-flop between opposite global time zones, fight to stay awake in the cockpit. Hospital interns drive themselves close to a delirious stupor while working shifts up to thirty hours straight. The once-sacred work ethic has become so distorted that worker burnout has created a huge and growing industry in legal gambling and lotteries. People are desperate to instantly hit the jackpot to break free from it all.

The Great Depression of the 1930s forced two professionals living in New York to ask fundamental questions about the rat race. Helen and Scott Nearing sought the elusive "good life" by rejecting regimented dependence on the industrial and consumer complex. Theirs was a "personal search for a simple, satisfying life on the land, to be devoted to mutual aid and harmlessness, with an ample margin of leisure in which to do personally constructive and creative work." They weren't seeking an escape from work: "Quite the contrary, we wanted to find a way in which we could put more into life and get more out of it. We were not shirking obligations but looking for an opportunity to take on more worthwhile responsibilities."[6]

The Nearings valued the work ethic in its purest sense—work-on-your-own-terms ethic. Their subsistence homesteading, not only largely freed them from the labor commodity markets, it also greatly freed their time for partaking of enriching pursuits and interests. "We were able to organize our work time so that six months of bread labor each year gave us six months of leisure, for research, traveling, writing, speaking and teaching."[7]

Their back-to-the-land and conservationist experiment was by no means easy, and the majority would likely find such self-sufficient living to be overly radical, harsh, and austere. For the Nearings, it turned out to be a highly satisfying and healthy way of life. For five decades they never had the need to visit a doctor, and both lived long lives; Scott died at age one hundred, and Helen might have lived as long had she not died in a car accident at age ninety-one.

The Nearings discovered for themselves a rewarding and autonomous formula for living that was similar to that adopted by hunter-gatherers and traditional indigenous subsistence cultures. Marshall Sahlins referred to such people as the "original affluent society," shattering common misconceptions about "primitive" living in his in-depth study of their economics.[8] At the most, adult workers in such cultures spent three to five hours per day in food production, a far cry from the hours punched in by workers earning their dough on modern civilization's treadmill. "Hunter-gatherers consume less energy per capita per year than any other group of human beings," Sahlins wrote. "Yet when you come to examine it the original affluent society was none other than the hunter's—in which all the people's material wants were easily satisfied. To accept that hunters are affluent is therefore to recognize that the present human condition of man slaving to bridge the gap between his unlimited wants and his insufficient means is a tragedy of modern times."[9]

There's no question that progress has improved our lives in many ways. Where I live in Canada, we have a climate of extremes; the temperature can rise to 40° Celsius (104° F) in the summer and dip to a very frosty minus 40° Celsius (minus 40° F) in the winter. During the depths of January, when a blizzard could be raging outside, I have a great appreciation for how progress makes my life a whole lot easier. It's very reassuring to have a furnace with natural gas piped in to keep our house warm at night. There are wonderful comforts when rising in the morning: a flush toilet, hot running water for a shower, electricity for lights and appliances, a refrigerator stocked full of food purchased at the nearby supermarket where the goods never run out. The comforts go on and on when you really stop to think of them. The Y2K scare a few years ago jarred many Canadians, because the thought of trying to survive in the winter without modern amenities was a frightening proposition.

Unfortunately, what was largely ignored when industrial progress was in its infancy was that, for every benefit or improvement, there would be a corresponding downside. Not everyone in the era of the industrial revolution was enthralled with the idea of mechanized progress. Some skeptics and dissenters were gravely concerned about losses amid the gains. Mary Shelley's classic novel, *Frankenstein,* warned in 1818 of the dangers of unleashing an industrialized monster that could turn against us. Our current ecological crisis, together with the amount of human slaughter every year in industry and transportation, are just two examples of her amazing foresight. Of course, those are unintentional forms of destruction—what have been either traditionally brushed aside or euphemistically called accidents.*

The road to hell was indeed paved with good intentions. The rat race isn't an evolutionary concept whereby getting ahead at all costs is in the cards. Even Charles Darwin was apparently bitter about his theory of evolution being distorted as "the law of the jungle" or "survival of the fittest" and then misused to justify all sorts of self-serving aggression.[10] Lewis Mumford noted how utopian dreams of a mechanized power system degraded into "poisonous effluents" among an affluent society.[11] Taoism warned of this danger many centuries before:

> Do you think you can take over the universe and
> improve it?

---

*Our roads are deadlier than the battlefields. During combat in the Second World War, almost three hundred thousand American soldiers were killed in the line of duty. With vehicle accidents now accounting for nearly forty-five thousand deaths each year in the United States, the last decade alone realized more fatalities than WWII.

I do not believe it can be done.
The universe is sacred.
You cannot improve it.
If you try to change it, you will ruin it.
If you try to hold it, you will lose it.[12]

As beneficiaries of the mess and misfortune we must deal with on the planet, we've learned the hard way that technology is far more damaging then ever envisioned. David Suzuki, a Canadian geneticist and long-time host of the television program *The Nature of Things,* contends, "There is no such thing as a problem-free technology." The difficulty with evaluating the pros and cons of new technology is that "the benefits . . . are always immediate and obvious," but the negative consequences are speculative at best. "We don't have the knowledge base to be able to predict precise [negative] consequences," he says, "and so we are stuck sounding vague."[13]

Physics teaches that for every action there is an equal and opposite reaction. The benefits gained by improved sanitation, rapid transportation, and plentiful supplies of food have been offset by the destructive influences of dependence on mechanization and technological gadgets. People aren't as healthy as was promised. Nutrition author and educator Herbert Shelton, an advocate of "natural hygiene" (lifestyle choices that help prevent disease), noted the consequences decades ago. "What we are pleased to call the 'progress of modern science' has been, in many ways, a health-destroying influence. . . . Our engineers have turned out myriads of labor-saving devices and these have been made to supercede the use and development of the powers of the body and mind."[14]

STRESS AND STRAIN

Terms such as *force, stress, strain, pressure,* and *tension* are part of our everyday language. Initially applied in the physical sciences and engineering, these terms were later adopted to describe human conditions. In the psychological sense, they usually refer to circumstances that are negative or unpleasant. People might speak of being forced to do something against their wishes, the stress of working tight deadlines at the office, the strain in grieving the loss of a loved one, the pressure before an important event, or the tension in a difficult marriage. Often these terms are used interchangeably and synonymously, and most people can probably relate to what they mean to each of us on a very personal level.

Stress is very broadly used nowadays to describe both an external situation—for example, a *stressful* job interview—and the resulting consequences to the individual—the person being interviewed feeling *stressed out* afterward. Technically, an external stress cannot be both a cause *and* an effect; rather, strain is the subsequent reaction to the stress. Dr. Hans Selye, the eminent physician who pioneered the concept of the general adaptation syndrome (GAS), also called the stress syndrome, said years later he'd erred in the use of the phrase *stress reaction*. He said he should have used the term *strain reaction*. Because stress had gained such widespread use in health circles by then, to avoid the confusion, he developed the name *stressor* to denote a stressful situation and *stress* the resulting adverse effect.[15] To be consistent with Bates's use of the term *strain* in his writings, I use the conventional terms and connotations: *stress* is an externally imposed cause, and *strain* is the effect on the individual. To be clear on the distinction, let's consider some examples, the first in the engineering sense and the others as applied to people.

When a person stands on the end of a diving board at the swimming pool, the board curves downward from the force of the person's body weight. The force spread over the cross-sectional area in the board is said be a stress. The deformation, or stretching, in the fibers at the support end of the board is said to be the resultant strain. The fibers pull and elongate (in tension) on the top from the weight, and if enough people were to get on the end, the board would continue to deform and curve downward. The strain in the board's top fibers at the support end of the board would keep increasing proportionally until it became too great. The board would no longer have the capacity to hold the weight, and the fibers would eventually rip and rupture, causing a collapse.

Now let's consider a similar concept, but in the human body. Two boxers are going at it in the ring when one lands a solid and forceful blow (stress) to the other's jaw. The boxer on the receiving end feels the result (strain) instantly in the form of feedback called pain. The muscles and bones strain under the stress, and the bone may break—the proverbial glass jaw. In this example, the force was clearly visible, at least to the spectators—if not to the recipient of the blow, who didn't see it coming! But what about a case where the force is invisible and self-inflicted?

Imagine a hypothetical student is studying a difficult subject and is worried about getting a passing grade. This particular student has an unconscious habit of clenching her jaw while concentrating hard, trying desperately to mentally grasp the facts. She eventually gets a severe headache in the attempt to store, assimilate, and recall all the information. Studying late into the evening, she reaches a stage where she can no longer absorb any more information. Although she's exhausted, she has trouble falling asleep—and when sleep finally comes, it's very fitful. During her sleep, the mental tension continues, and she loudly grinds her teeth. When she wakes in the morning, her jaw aches and so does her head. She reaches for the aspirin bottle to help numb the pain.

The stress in the student's case is the pressure imposed by the demands of the educational system. Unlike the boxer's fist, the force that initiates the stress cannot be seen per se, but the resulting strain and pain is very real, leading to physical harm. The invisible stress that causes mental or emotional strain affects us all in some way, shape, or form. In many cases, the damage resulting from the strain can ultimately have lethal consequences, and that is why stress has been dubbed the "silent killer."

HEALTH RISKS

Stress is the very stuff of life. A normal level of stress, both physically and mentally, is necessary for good health. Otherwise we'd be physically atrophied and mentally bored to pieces. In fact, without any stress, you'd be dead as a doornail. The essential and healthy level of stress is called *eustress*. But like anything, it can be too much of a good thing.

Balance is the key, for too much stress can spell trouble, especially if it is continual and prolonged. That's when it turns to *distress,* the unhealthy form of stress.

Researchers have recognized that there are many events in life that can cause distress, and they've even attempted to quantify them. The Holmes-Rahe Social Readjustment Rating Scale was developed in 1967 to help people gauge the stress levels in their lives. On the bottom of the scale, minor violation of the law counts for 10 points, while at the top of the scale, death of spouse counts 100. Somewhere in the middle of the pack a career change counts 36 points. The theory is that if your total score for the past year exceeds 150 points, then you have too much stress in your life. The chart is intended to be sort of a barometer or early-warning system. Recognize the potential danger level of stress, and then take action to try to reduce it. This theory assumes that everybody reacts with similar mental strain to stressful events in much the same way. But is this actually the case? For some adventure seekers, potentially stressful events are viewed as challenges to be overcome, the very spice of life. Many such people refer to themselves as adrenaline junkies—they seem to thrive living on the edge. Just consider the popularity of extreme sports nowadays and the rash of reality-TV programs, such as *Fear Factor,* that cater to people wanting to continually push the envelope. These people are highly competitive and hate to lose. They still feel fear, but they find it invigorating and motivating. But for many others, the exact same stressful situations would be unbearable. They would be absolutely gripped with terror and unable to carry through with the demands put before them.

"Sticks and stones may break my bones, but names can never hurt me" is much easier said than practiced. In highly charged situations, it's extremely challenging to maintain control of your mental state so as to keep the negative emotions in check. Just consider the politics of hate, rage, and revenge of warring factions throughout various regions of the world. It's a vicious cycle that just never seems to end from one generation to the next, averting any opportunity for peaceful resolutions.

The impact of strain from one person to the next, then, can be quite variable and difficult to predict. But regardless of individual thresholds, continually distressing circumstances pose serious health risks to everyone. In Great Britain, *The Health and Safety Executive* published guidelines for employers warning about the ill effects of work-related stress. A stressful work environment and the subsequent mental strain can have adverse physical effects on an employee, "such as raised heart rate, increased sweating, headache, dizziness, *blurred vision* [emphasis added], aching neck and shoulders, skin rashes and a lowering of risk to infection."[16] Indeed, several diseases are now known to be either caused by stress or worsened by stress. Categories include cardiovascular, gastrointestinal, neurological, and immune disorders.

Researchers had once thought that stress played a role in a few diseases. As the list grows each year, it appears as though Selye was prophetic, having noted that "stress plays some role in the development of every disease."[17] The weakening of the immune system caused by stress is now believed to have another lethal impact. Although the exact causes of cancer, probably the most dreaded disease that continues to plague humankind, aren't fully understood, stress is suspected to play a role. It is now theorized that a weakened immune system encourages the development of cancerous cells.[18]

But it's not just physical disorders and ailments that accumulate from life's stresses. The British guidelines to employers also lists adverse behavioral effects, "such as increased anxiety and irritability, a tendency to drink more alcohol and smoke more, difficulty sleeping, poor concentration and an inability to deal calmly with everyday tasks and situations."[19] Mental health statistics seem to bear out the notion that we are driving ourselves mad in the "chase and hunt." Here is a sampling of the sobering data to give an indication of how widespread the problem is among the general public in the United States:[20]

- 58 million Americans ages 18 and older—about one in four adults—suffer from a diagnosable mental disorder in a given year.
- Major depressive disorder (depression) affects 15 million American adults age 18 and older every year.

- Over 30,000 people die by suicide annually in the United States, and more than 90 percent of those have a diagnosable mental disorder.
- Roughly 40 million American adults ages 18 and older have an anxiety disorder such as panic disorder, obsessive-compulsive disorder or phobias.
- Eating disorders (anorexia nervosa, bulimia nervosa, binge-eating disorder) impact millions of teens and young women annually.
- Mental disorders are the leading cause of disability in the United States and Canada for ages 15–44.

With stress, physical and behavioral symptoms are wed. As in the old ditty about love and marriage, you can't have one without the other. For example, depression greatly increases the risk of developing heart disease. Depressed people are at four times greater risk of a heart attack than those who have no history of depression.[21] A person with an obsessive-compulsive disorder may also suffer a gastrointestinal problem that requires medical attention. The combined physical and behavioral reactions can become very pronounced after exposure to more severe stress.

The most acute form of stress-related illness now recognized by mental health professionals is called post-traumatic stress disorder (PTSD). According to the National Institute of Mental Health, PTSD "is an anxiety disorder that can develop after exposure to a terrifying event or ordeal in which grave physical harm occurred or was threatened. Traumatic events that may trigger PTSD include violent personal assaults, natural or human-caused disasters, accidents, or military combat." Sufferers of PTSD remain haunted by the original trauma, continually reliving the horror. "Many people with PTSD repeatedly re-experience the ordeal in the form of flashback episodes, memories, nightmares, or frightening thoughts, especially when they are exposed to events or objects reminiscent of the trauma. Anniversaries of the event can also trigger symptoms."[22]

A television documentary told the story of Canadian soldiers who suffered PTSD after a peacekeeping mission in the war-torn region of Bosnia. The Canadian soldiers were not in the heat of battle but were helping search for possible survivors of "ethnic cleansing." Instead, they found the victims—men, women, and children—massacred and buried in shallow graves. The job of the peacekeepers all of a sudden became that of morticians, exhuming corpses and transporting them to a morgue for identification. The young men were clearly neither trained nor emotionally conditioned for what they encountered. During one interview, a soldier tearfully recounted the shock of dealing with a teenage girl's decomposing body; the heat was enough to melt the rubber gloves the soldiers were wearing.

Upon their return to Canada, the soldiers began displaying classic symptoms of PTSD and had trouble coping with civilian and home life. Many suffered from such problems as insomnia, depression, sharp mood swings, and intense anger at inappropriate times. Some also developed physical afflictions such as joint disorders and digestive problems. One peacekeeper's PTSD physical problem really caught my attention, though. It turned out he was slowly *going blind in one eye.*

The day-to-day grind is obviously not as acute a stressor as a situation that causes PTSD. Nevertheless, the results of the strain accumulate and are quite serious. The data on physical and mental illness from the workplace could be viewed from another angle, however: perhaps they signify a symptom of human *health,* not disease. The diagnosis may be misplaced; does the sickness rest within society itself? The rash of health problems is a strong message that we have a huge imbalance in our hurried and harried lifestyles. Noteworthy among the health problems is the general decline of visual acuity in industrialized nations. We will explore this loss next.

2
Loss

Force is followed by loss of strength.
This is not the way of Tao.

Calculated sharpness
cannot be kept for long.

Lao Tzu[1]

Cyclops, the one-eyed giant of Greek mythology, would make a good poster boy for technological progress. His characteristics parallel the many values and outcomes of an industrial society: he is colossal in size, power, and strength; wild and insolent in destroying the planet; and he devours humans with deadly and risky technology. To modernize Cyclops, simply have him clutching steroids in one hand and amphetamines in another, thus symbolizing addictions with no regard to limits: further bloated growth and unending speed. But the most fitting representation has to be Cyclops's single eye focusing solely on the benefits of progress.

The single-eyed approach to vision care—treating only symptoms of defective sight—has dominated the scene for quite some time. As writer Aldous Huxley pointed out, the orthodox method "has been carried to a high degree of perfection, and, within its limitations, is reasonably successful."[2] By "successful," he meant the quick fix of artificial lenses that permits most wearers to function rather well with their aid. But, it's the limitations that are disconcerting and should not be swept aside as merely nuisance factors. The treatment itself is a large part of the problem. Ironically, the visual health of the populace has lost ground since the advent of vision science and the outcome has been an "incalculable amount of human misery" as Bates so lucidly predicted over eighty years ago. This chapter addresses the miseries.

CIVILIZED VISION

Those at the forefront of industrialized civilizations had no reason to believe, or likely even suspect, that the new way of life would have any adverse impact on people's eyesight. After all, it was a highly optimistic time with dreams of a mechanistic society, perfectly synchronized. Yet, as more people than ever before in the civilized world were becoming literate, it wasn't long before a large percentage of them began to have vision problems. There was no escaping the fact that the vision of industrialized people had declined substantially. The modernized countries had to continually lower their vision standards for their armies, otherwise too many potential recruits would have been rejected.[3]

The troubling aspect of the massive vision problem was that the great inventive minds of the day, with all their technological wizardry, could not find a way of stopping what had become an epidemic. By the turn of the twentieth century, Bates noted that the medical profession had for over a hundred years "been seeking for some method of checking the ravages of civilization upon the human eye."[4] After pouring large sums of money into research investigating the cause, the specialists were no farther ahead than when they started. So they essentially just threw their arms in the air, so to speak, and concluded they could do nothing more. They suggested it was simply the price to be paid for a civilized way of life.

This conclusion did not sit well in the least with Bates: "We are told," he wrote, "that for these [visual] ills, which are not only so inconvenient, but often so distressing and dangerous, there is not only no cure, and no palliatives save those optic crutches known as eyeglasses, but, under modern conditions of life, practically no prevention." In other words, the only thing to do was to keep prescribing glasses for all different types of blurry sight. Much like the military, industrialized society couldn't afford to lose recruits needed for its factories and offices.

Because the members of the orthodoxy believed they could do no more, they firmly concluded that the human eye was not adapted to a civilized society. The eye had supposedly evolved mainly for distance vision in the preindustrial role of hunter, herdsman, farmer, or fighter and could not withstand the unnatural demands of a literate society. But Bates pointed out, "The fact that primitive woman was a seamstress, an embroiderer, a weaver, an artist in all sorts of fine and beautiful work, appears to have been generally forgotten. Yet women living under primitive conditions have just as good eyesight as the men."[5] Bates also noted, "The lower animals when subjected to civilized conditions respond to them in precisely the same way as do human creatures. I have examined many domestic and menagerie animals, and have found them, in many cases, myopic, although they neither read, nor write, nor sew, nor set type."[6]

Statistics paint a sorry picture of the state of eyesight in civilized society—certainly not one of progress, but of continual degeneration and increasing morbidity. In traditional cultures lacking literacy and intellectual pursuits, but rich in oral language and art, myopia is virtually nonexistent. As well, only 2 to 3 percent of children in North America are born with visual deformities. Yet the rate of myopia in industrialized nations has increased over the years to rather alarming numbers, as reported by optometrist Richard Kavner in 1979: "Before age 10 approximately four to six percent of the population is nearsighted. By the time children are through the eighth grade, 20 percent are nearsighted. At the end of high school the number has jumped to 40 percent. And throughout college the number varies from 60 to 80 percent, with the higher percentages among the honors and graduate students."[7]

It is ironic that, while Western society is gradually adopting more

Eastern approaches to healing and medicine, Japan, China, Singapore, Taiwan, and Korea now have a skyrocketing dependence on the use of optical wares. The incidence of myopia in those countries can be said to be of epidemic proportions, far surpassing the North American numbers. It's the same pattern; both the prevalence and severity of myopia are higher as the level of education increases. They're paying a steep price for the manic, competitive pace. In 1999, Japan reported myopia rates of 30 percent at age eleven, 50 percent at age fifteen, and 70 percent by age seventeen.[8] Taiwan was found to have the highest incidence of myopia among schoolchildren, an astounding 85 percent![9]

There are also many people in civilized society who are farsighted, unable to read without the aid of glasses. A significant proportion of the population is inflicted with this type of visual blur, perhaps as high as 50 percent in the West.[10]

With so many people having vision difficulties, whether near or far, the "correction" industry is obviously very substantial. It certainly hasn't abated since Aldous Huxley's day, when he said, "The manufacture of optical glass is now a considerable industry, and its retail sale a profitable branch of commerce."[11] The vision-care industry accumulated an astounding $25.7 billion in revenues for the twelve-month period ending March 2005, in large part thanks to the 147 million American adults who depend on prescription eyewear. That's 66 percent of the adult population who regularly pay for eye exams and new, trendy glasses. The refractive surgery (eye surgery to correct blurred vision, such as laser eye surgery) sector also accounts for a piece of the massive revenues, as costs range from $1,000 to $2,500 per eye depending on the procedure.

It comes as no surprise that this sector—close to two million surgeries undertaken annually in the United States—is enjoying the greatest market growth, up 46 percent from the previous year. In comparison, the next highest growth sectors during the same period were for the sale of reading glasses and contact lenses, up 14 percent and 4 percent respectively.[12]

"EYE"-ATROGENESIS

The notion that medical practices may be bad for your health was mainly unknown a generation ago. The concept of *iatrogenesis,* damage inadvertently inflicted in the course of medical treatment, came into prominence after the groundbreaking exposé by Ivan Illich in *Limits to Medicine: Medical Nemesis, the Expropriation of Health* in the mid-1970s. The topic is now in the forefront when the Institute of Medicine, part of the Academy of Sciences, confirms that medical errors are a leading cause of death.[13] Similarly, the Centers for Disease Control and Prevention has published data on the alarming spread of infectious diseases in hospitals.[14]

Medical consumers are much more informed nowadays. The explosive popularity of alternative and complementary modalities is evidence of a growing dissatisfaction with and distrust of invasive and technological treatments. In fields of medicine other than those specializing in the eye, a significant sector of the population is turning more toward alternative and complementary solutions. Four out of ten Americans are now choosing more natural therapies for chronic conditions such as anxiety, back problems, neck problems, and headaches.[15]

Although the public is more aware of the risks of traditional medicine, little do people realize the extent of clinical iatrogenesis in the eye-care industry. No matter what the treatment for blurred vision—whether it is glasses, contact lenses, or some type of refractive surgery—there are negative consequences. Let's consider each of these three categories.

Glasses

Children who are prescribed glasses for myopia have no idea of the long-term consequences and damage that result from their continual wear. As consumers of curative eye-care, their parents believe they are doing the right thing in providing their children with the benefits of artificially clear sight. Most children find, as I did, that once they begin to wear glasses, and wear them continually, their vision gets worse. Stronger lenses are prescribed, usually each year, until the condition stabilizes at some point. For some, the end result can be powerful prescription lenses. Bates wrote:

> Eyeglasses . . . always do more or less harm, and at their best they never improve the vision to normal. . . . That glasses must injure the eye is evident. . . . It means that [the wearer] is maintaining constantly a degree of refractive error which otherwise would not be maintained constantly. It is only to be expected that this should make the condition worse, and it is a matter of common experience that it does. After people once begin to wear glasses their strength, in most cases, has to be steadily increased in order to maintain the degree of visual acuity secured by the aid of the first pair. . . . We have the testimony of Dr. Sidler-Huguenin, of Zurich, that of the thousands of myopes [nearsighted people] treated by him the majority grew steadily worse, in spite of all the skill he could apply to the fitting of glasses for them.[16]

This is one of the critical distinctions between what Bates believed and what the orthodoxy preached. Bates maintained that myopia worsened as children strained to adapt to the glasses—an iatrogenic outcome. The orthodoxy, on the other hand, preferred to invent a disorder that was either a result of genetics (an abnormally long eyeball), the environment (too much close work), or a combination of both. They called the phenomenon *progressive myopia*.

The old theory persists to this day. I have seen recent optometric marketing information stating that progressive myopia can only be corrected by glasses. It suggests that frequent prescription changes do not make the eyes weaker, asserting that the blur continues to get worse as the child goes through a rapid growth period. Such children, supposedly doomed by hereditary factors, must be prescribed glasses to keep up with the changes. In my own case, this line of thinking is bogus. My progressive myopia progressively reversed and diminished once I rid myself of glasses and began using my eyes naturally again.

Nearsighted people have better visual acuity under bright light, so glasses prescribed for poorer indoor lighting are automatically too strong outside. More than once I can remember wearing my glasses for the first time after they were fitted with an upgraded prescription. After stepping outside the optometrist's office into the brighter, natural light of the sun, I recall just how dizzy I felt. The sidewalk beneath my feet was so wild! Everything looked much different as I walked, and I had to be careful not to trip. In hindsight, I realize now that the glasses were far too powerful under those conditions. But I faithfully wore them, not questioning authority. I figured the glasses must have been proper; so, like many kids with glasses, I got used to them. Within a few days, things started to look and feel normal again. I've since theorized that my eyes rapidly deteriorated in those first few days to adjust to overly powerful lenses—it didn't take a year for the next checkup to confirm the further loss of acuity.

The other variable that makes nearsighted glasses too strong is the distance objects are viewed from the eyes. Optometrist Joseph Kennebeck explained that nearsighted glasses are prescribed for just one distance—twenty feet. Glass is rigid, so looking through the lenses at objects closer than twenty feet means the eyes have to overaccommodate (unnaturally strain to adjust focus) because the glasses are too strong for close work. This is referred to as *near-point stress*. Kennebeck contended that there was a direct relationship between the distance and the stress: "At TEN feet the glasses are TWICE wrong; at FIVE feet the glasses are FOUR times wrong; at ONE foot, where all close work is done, the glasses are TWENTY times wrong. . . . The eyes cannot compensate . . . WITHOUT BEING HURT. It is the compensating, through myopic glasses fitted for twenty feet, that brings on progressive myopia."[17] Huxley stated that wearing glasses "confines the eyes to a state of rigid and unvarying structural immobility" and compared them to "splints, iron braces and plaster casts."[18]

Many other forward-thinking optometrists and eye doctors have also agreed on the iatrogenic consequence of glasses. In fact, an entire new field of the profession—behavioral optometry—has evolved to help prevent or diminish progressive myopia in children, and one of the strategies developed is to prescribe bifocals. The more powerful upper portion of the lens is for looking at distant objects; the much weaker lower portion is for close work, thus reducing the near-point stress.

When I was in about grade six, I had bifocals prescribed by an optometrist who was obviously concerned about the progression of my myopia. Knowing I was dependent on glasses, he was hoping to at least try and halt the problem. But a few months later, our family moved to another community, and I received my next checkup from a different optometrist, one from the "old school." I remember him telling my parents that it was ridiculous for me to be wearing bifocals, "They're only meant for older people, not children," he declared, essentially ridiculing the other optometrist's actions. My parents trusted his judgment, so my next pair of stronger glasses was the "full meal deal," thus completely thwarting the efforts of the first optometrist to prevent the cycle of further damage.

Concave (minus) lenses used to compensate for myopia have been called "poison" by others. Even before Bates's time, young men in Russia wanting to evade conscription in the army during the 1800s apparently knew their damaging effects. In his book *Spectacle Hobby*, optometrist Jacob Raphaelson noted, "A few months before . . . the conscript went to an optical doctor and got a pair of strong minus glasses which he wore steadily until prior to the [military eye] examination. He was then sure that he would be rejected on account of his vision. The minus glasses had weakened his eyes and made his distant vision very poor."[19]

Neville Schuller, a vision specialist in Toronto, said in 1938, "I would like to have a law established forbidding the prescribing of minus glasses without extenuating circumstances."[20] Optometrist Samuel Druker wrote in 1946, "The suspicion began to dawn on me slowly that among the causes of progressive myopia it might be necessary to list concave (minus) lenses themselves. From many articles that have appeared in the past on the subject of 'Optical Poison,' a familiar term a decade ago, many other optometrists appear to have the same idea."[21]

More recently, behavioral optometrist Roberto Kaplan wrote in a similar vein that strong myopic lenses create a dependency "which is as insidious in its own way as a dependency on sugar, drugs, or alcohol. . . . I really believed that recommending full-strength lens prescriptions for my patients would help their eyes to 'get better.' After working with thousands of patients . . . I realized that I was actually contributing to their vision loss."[22]

The next stage beyond myopia is even more disconcerting. Many now concur with Bates that, once myopia advances to a high degree, more serious disorders can potentially develop, leading to permanent vision loss. These conditions include:

- Cataracts—the lens in the eye becomes cloudy or opaque.
- Glaucoma—fluid pressure inside the eye rises and places stress on the optic nerve.
- Detached retina—the light receptive layer at the back of the eye begins to tear loose.
- Macular degeneration—the central vision becomes diseased.

Various organizational and government statistics gathered on the incidence of blindness verify that the leading cause of these serious vision disorders is myopia. Optometrist Maurice Brumer stated in a paper presented at a scientific conference in 1979:

The complications of myopia are numerous and grave, frequently resulting in blindness. The degenerative changes appear typically in adult life after the myopia has been fully established for some years. . . . Few [myopic] people, faced with the prospect of blindness in old age, realize that their problems actually began in childhood when they were first fitted with the first pair of corrective (negative) lenses by someone who was probably unconcerned about the tragic, long-term results of that action. Few of these people realize how their situation became more precarious each time their glasses were strengthened and nothing was said about prevention. Now, when it is too late for prevention, they find themselves in the hands of surgeons who are making their living from someone else's mistakes by trying to patch up steadily deteriorating retinas. The patient has been a lifelong victim of ignorance and exploitation.[23]

An estimated 2.7 million Canadians suffer severe vision impairment, being either legally blind or having low-vision status. That's over 10 percent of the population. Legally blind is defined as best visual acuity with prescription lenses of 20/200* or worse in the better eye, or a visual field that is restricted to 20 degrees or less. Low vision is defined as best visual acuity with prescription lenses in the range of 20/60 to 20/200. At the end of 2002, statistics for those legally blind showed the following prevalence by age group:[24]

- 5 percent age seventeen and under;
- 8 percent ages eighteen to forty-nine;
- 13 percent ages fifty to sixty-nine; and
- 74 percent age seventy and over.

The natural response to these data is to conclude vision loss is an inevitable consequence of aging. But is it? Is this degree of vision impairment in the elderly population perhaps due to phase three of the general adaptation syndrome (GAS) noted earlier? The GAS *triphasic response* to distress, according to Hans Selye, is "1) the alarm reaction; 2) the stage of resistance; and 3) the stage of exhaustion."[25] At first, he says, the distressful experience "is difficult, then one gets used to it, and finally one cannot stand it any longer."[26]

---

*In 1864, Dutch ophthalmologist Herman Snellen set the 20/20 standard for normal eyesight. The Snellen chart is the one with the big letter "E" at the top, and rows of letters which get smaller and smaller toward the bottom. Depending on the size of the chart, the big "E" in the top row may be the "100 line" and the bottom row with the smallest sized letters may be the "10 line." A person seeing no better than the 100 line from 20 feet is said to have 20/100 vision. The first number designates the distance the person stands from the chart and the second number designates the lowest row that can be read. One who can read all the letters in the "10 line" from 20 feet away will have 20/10 vision, keener than normal acuity. That person would be able to read the top 100 line standing a distance of 200 feet away.

When a young person develops myopia, has the child perhaps gone through an initial alarm phase? If so, the blur could be thought of as a symptom that is superficial at this point. That is to say, the myopia is a temporary demand on the eyes caused by stress and is reversible relatively quickly if caught soon enough through NVI relaxation methods. If the myopia is not reversed by NVI, another alarm stage hits at the first wearing of prescription lenses to neutralize the blur.

When a child gets glasses for myopia, the initial tension responsible for the blur is never addressed and now is sure to be maintained. The glasses feel weird and produce such reactions as headaches, dizziness, or slight nausea. But in the second phase of the GAS, the body eventually blocks out these reactions and the person gets used to the lenses. It may take a few years for this stage of adaptation to plateau as the child gets progressively stronger lenses. The symptom of blur is no longer superficial but deeply ingrained at this point.

If people continue wearing their prescription lenses faithfully through adulthood, as most do, does this second GAS phase continue until it reaches a point in retirement years when the eyes scream out, "That's it! We can't take this tension any more! Enough is enough!"? Maybe the eyes' capacity for continuous adaptation to stress is finally depleted, reaching the third GAS phase of exhaustion. If so, permanent vision impairment may ensue. The golden years of freedom could become the darkened years of despair and dependence.

Contact Lenses

Contact lenses cause much the same damage as that outlined for glasses, but they have more harmful effects that can be added to the list. NVI instructor Tom Quackenbush says, "The painful 'adaptation' period experienced by wearers of hard contact lenses is a message to stop putting foreign objects into the eyes!"[27] Some of the iatrogenic problems people have experienced with lenses are:

- Sudden pain and dizziness;
- Distortion of the cornea;

- Irritation of the eyes and eyelids;
- Cornea abrasions, infections, ulcers, or inflammation;
- Drying out of the eyes;
- Oxygen deprivation of the eyes; and
- Vision loss.

When I first got contact lenses, my optometrist warned me about the danger of being outside during windy days when the dust kicked up. He knew from firsthand experience, so he gave me some pointers on what to do. If a piece of dust were to get caught in between my eye and the contact lens, he said I'd know right away by the intense pain and tearing. When it happened, I would have to remove the lens as quickly as possible, or the speck of dust would damage the cornea. He showed me how to cup one hand over my eye while the other hand was underneath popping out the lens with a finger. The idea was to huddle away from the wind to prevent the lens from blowing away. Sure enough, one dusty day the intense pain and tearing was unmistakable. I managed to save the lens as I was taught in the office lesson. I got used to dreading windy days and had to perform the technique many times.

There was another time when my contact lenses were driving me crazy with irritation, so I went to see the optometrist. He checked my eyes and found some minor damage occurring to my corneas. He asked what I was using for a lens-cleaning and -soaking solution. I told him the brand I'd been using up till then was sold out, so I ended up getting another product. He figured the irritation was caused by an allergic reaction to the new solution. I had to find the old brand at another store, and once I changed back, the problem subsided. I was lucky, for more serious complications can result from contact lens solutions.

The Centers for Disease Control and Prevention (CDC) reports that wearers of soft contact lenses are at risk of contracting *microbial keratitis,* a severe infection of the cornea. Those at greatest risk are wearers of overnight lenses. Symptoms of microbial keratitis include unusual redness, eye pain, tearing, discharge, sensitivity to light, blurry vision, or swelling. Although the risk of contracting microbial keratitis is low (an incidence of 4 to 21 cases per 10,000), serious cases that don't respond to medications usually require surgery. A corneal transplant is necessary in the most severe cases where permanent vision loss results.[28]

Early in 2006, the CDC began receiving data that suggested a greater incidence of *fungal keratitis,* a type of microbial keratitis, occurred among soft contact wearers. As many as 130 cases of the fungal infection were under investigation in several states throughout the United States. The CDC determined that the majority of those infected were using particular brands of contact lens solution. At the early stage in the investigation, the CDC had full data available for thirty cases; of those, eight patients required corneal transplants.[29]

These keratitis cases prompted both the Food and Drug Administration (FDA) and the CDC to issue public warnings. In addition, the manufacturer of the soft contact lens solutions voluntarily withdrew their particular products from the marketplace to conduct an internal investigation. They, too, issued a public statement warning people to immediately stop using the products identified by the CDC. The public statements also cautioned people to be vigilant of proper hygienic practices for the use and care of lenses and solutions.

Refractive Surgery

Refractive surgery, the latest high-tech "cure" for blurry vision, comes in many types, all with unique acronyms: LASIK, LASEK, PRK, RK, AK, ALK. There's no need to explain the technical differences, because whether the eyes are cut with a scalpel or laser beam, the net outcome for many is harm and pain.

Doctors touted the risks as minimal when the various refractive surgical procedures were introduced as "cutting edge" (literally!), because the long-term consequences were unknown. Prospective patients believed the marketing brochures and felt confident the high-tech surgeries were low risk. Pandora's box is wide open now. As reported in the United Kingdom, "Laser eye clinics are misleading customers by claiming that the operation is virtually risk-free when in fact one in 10 operations fail. Glossy brochures and websites which quote post-surgery 'complication' rates as low as just one in 1,000 do not mention that up to 10 percent of patients will have to have further surgery."[30]

Here we return to the discussion of overstating technological benefits while downplaying risks. Applied science is fraught with poor or inadequate risk assessment; not even the esteemed NASA organization was immune from such shortcomings. As acclaimed physicist Richard Feynman concluded in his report on the 1986 *Challenger* space shuttle disaster,* "For a successful technology, reality must take precedence over public relations, for nature cannot be fooled."[31] The reality of refractive surgery is clear now; nature has called the bluff. Scores of people have found out the hard way that the risks of damage to the delicate eyeball were greater than anticipated.

From a percentage perspective, the risks of serious consequences from refractive surgery may sound low, perhaps "only" 2 or 3 percent. But those are poor odds from an absolute-number standpoint. For every million surgeries undertaken per year, twenty to thirty thousand people are victimized. In response to the high numbers affected, an organization called Surgical Eyes was founded. As its Web site states, "It is the responsibility of the refractive surgical community finally to come to grips with the importance of using new methods to evaluate outcomes. . . . We have garnered the attention of the medical community, as a real and growing segment of the post-refractive surgical patient population, not isolated misadventures, but rather as a coherent group that shows similar patterns of visual symptoms and manifestations."[32]

Research reports describing unsatisfactory patient outcomes have come to the forefront in the past several years. Many patients haven't received the perfect vision they expected. Some have had to resort to glasses again, while others deal with annoying and permanent diffi-

---

*Two and a half years after the *Challenger* report, risk expert Harold Lewis reported that NASA hadn't made any significant changes in its safety protocol once the shuttle program resumed. From a probabilistic risk assessment (PRA) standpoint, he saw the dangers as too great. Although he dearly hoped otherwise, the odds showed him there was "no persuasive reason to believe" future missions would be free from another catastrophic failure (*Technological Risk*, 106). Sadly, the *Columbia* mission confirmed his fears.

culties for which prescription lenses cannot compensate. Surgical Eyes lists seventy-six possible complications of refractive surgery in alphabetical order, from "aniseikonia (difference in image size between the two eyes)" to "vitreous detachment (floaters)."* It also lists four other "future induced difficulties," presumably complications that have a delayed onset.[33]

For moral support, the organization encourages people to write about their experiences in a group forum, and the online feedback is replete with stories of anguish and frustration. One entry in the forum exemplified how the preoperative dream of clear vision was shattered postoperatively. The patient's vision took many weeks to stabilize; then she found three months later that she needed an "enhancement" refractive procedure. She suffers symptoms of haze, regression, loss of contrast, dry eyes, ghosting, and double vision. A year after the operation, she needed to continue taking steroids to help stabilize her vision. If she discontinued the medication, she had to wear glasses to compensate for the blur. Driving at night was painful, and working at a computer for eight hours each day was a struggle. She felt her independence gradually slipping away; she was moving closer to work so she didn't have to drive. The most amazing part of this story was that the eye clinic judged her case to be a successful outcome.[34]

While such victims of current refractive surgery are struggling with their debilitating and irreversible outcomes, the industry is excitedly researching new surgical procedures for *presbyopia* ("old age" sight). Presbyopia, much like the myth of myopia, was invented as an inevitable disorder people develop once they reach middle age. Their aging eyes are supposed to deteriorate naturally to the stage where they become dependent on reading glasses. It's jokingly called the "short arm" syndrome: the arms aren't long enough to place reading material far enough away to see it clearly. Many people never get the condi-

---

*The "floaters" in this case refer to a serious condition, not the benign protein deposit floaters within the eyes that can sometimes be seen drifting in front of one's field of vision.

tion, and numerous others have reversed it naturally, including Bates himself.

One new surgical procedure involves using a probe to apply radio waves in a circular pattern to the outer periphery of the eye. The effect, which shrinks peripheral fibrous tissue, is similar to a band tightening the cornea to give it more curvature. In another procedure, plastic segments are permanently inserted in the eye to help give the lens more focusing curvature. Clinical trials typically involve a few patients whose outcomes are tracked over a couple of years or so.

These types of procedures seem to have no trouble passing the stringent approval processes of the appropriate agencies overseeing public health and safety. Yet what about safety five, ten, or twenty years from now? Researchers don't have a crystal ball that allows them to confidently extrapolate short-term data. The allure of science and technology combined with the profit motive—these techniques come with a hefty price tag—is just so overpowering that potential long-term iatrogenic outcomes are only marginally considered. Foreign pieces permanently implanted in the eyes, continually applying stress, surely has to signal unfavorable long-term consequences. A whole new category of victims' stories will most likely be added to the Surgical Eyes forum in the years to come.

AN ALTERNATIVE

Dr. Bates was a distinguished ophthalmologist, medical lecturer, and researcher in the late 1800s and early 1900s. As an eye surgeon, he also operated on many diseased or injured eyes. Early in his career he actually once prescribed glasses as the standard treatment of the day for nonpathological vision blur. Through years of experience he eventually concluded that poor eyesight generally resulted from the excesses of an overly industrialized and mechanized society. Furthermore, he found that the technology of prescription lenses actually exacerbated visual ills.

Bates ventured into territory that was essentially alien to his counterparts. He studied the role of mental and emotional strain on vision and came up with some very surprising findings. This led him to search for natural means to prevent, reverse, and alleviate the problem of blurred vision that had evaded medical science to that point.

Although improving eyesight naturally is still largely an underground practice, it is gradually gaining more widespread recognition. Others have taken over where Bates left off. The Association of Vision Educators is an organization based largely on his work. Its mission is "to increase public awareness of natural and integrated vision care and encourage education, communication and research in the field."[35] Its members include Bates Vision teachers, Natural Vision teachers, behavioral optometrists, and even some ophthalmologists. Another similar group, the Bates Association for Vision Education (BAVE), consists of "professionals dedicated to the teaching of vision improvement."[36]

The holistic method of NVI—instructing people to see in a more relaxed manner—is, as it turns out, in tune with the Tao. Part 2 explains how the fundamentals of NVI are truly the Way.

PART TWO

THE WAY

Tao follows what is natural.
LAO TZU

3
RHYTHM

So creatures sometimes go and sometimes follow,
sometimes puff and sometimes blow,
are sometimes strong and sometimes weak,
begin sometime and end sometime.

Controlling the breath causes strain.
If too much energy is used, exhaustion follows.
This is not the way of Tao.

LAO TZU[1]

Do you like music? Regardless of individual tastes, I would have to think that everyone is moved by some style of music. If ever there was a universal language that sweeps across boundaries, cultural groups, generation gaps, and historical eras, surely it is song. The beat and rhythm of a musical composition somehow connects to our primal instincts, evoking a wide range of emotions and feelings. It's hard not to tap your feet or sway along with an uplifting favorite song. Melodramatic songs can give us goose bumps or make us cry. From bygone days to contemporary trends, our vocabulary abounds with such mood-resonating genres and styles as ragtime, boogie woogie, swing, bebop, blues, rock and roll, soul, funk, heavy metal, and hip-hop. Is it any wonder, then, that when we are in agreement or congruence with someone, we use such metaphors as "singing from the same song sheet," "being on the same wavelength," and "getting good vibes"?

Taoism embraces many virtues centered on nature and plant life, such as rhythm, softness, flexibility, and yielding. These virtues parallel the teachings of NVI. This chapter outlines how our eyes love rhythm, vibrating to their own unique tempo as they absorb their surroundings. We also discuss how strain negatively impacts the natural rhythm. These two core findings—the ebb and flow of eyesight, and the effect of stress on vision—serve as the very foundation of the Bates Method and NVI.

CYCLICAL NATURE

The sun rises and sets. The moon changes from new to full. The ocean tide crests and recedes. Winter, spring, summer, and autumn go round and round. We sleep and wake, inhale and exhale, eat and excrete. The stock market swings from bullish to bearish. Athletes have peaks and slumps. The continual cycles of the universe, the earth, and all nature's life forms were observed and revered by ancient civilizations long before clocks were invented. The famous biblical passage from Ecclesiastes recognized this very cyclical nature of life: "To every thing there is a season, and a time to every purpose under the heaven." The Taoist excerpts at the beginning of this chapter echo these cyclical workings, which, as Ellen Chen observes, are "always in the process of change: rising or falling, coming out or going back. . . . The sage is sensitive to the rhythm of the world and follows its contours of change."[2]

The related Eastern dualist concept of yin/yang, which is becoming a household term in Western society these days, also embraces the importance of being in tune with rhythms. The symbol for yin/yang—curved and fluid black and white shapes embracing and flowing together within a circle—represents the unending pattern of reversal from one state to another in a cyclical manner. Rather than fixed, absolute, and competing opposites, these states are flexible, changing, and complementary. Again, from the Tao Te Ching:

Therefore having and not having arise together.
Difficult and easy complement each other.
Long and short contrast each other;
High and low rest upon each other;
Voice and sound harmonize each other;
Front and back follow one another.[3]

Modern society has recently rediscovered the importance of life's rhythms. Chronobiology is a "new wave" of scientific and medical research that has emerged to study the rhythmic cycles of humans. Carol Orlock explains:

Chronobiology reveals how life—the biology of all living things—inscribes patterns in time. Every human being . . . is a finely tuned system of many interlocking inner clocks, each displaying a distinct rhythm. Because the concept of time is built into us at the cellular level, biological clocks . . . dictate our desires and disinclinations, moods, hungers, abilities and vulnerabilities. . . . Applications from this new science are arriving in nearly every realm of modern life, from architecture and engineering to law and the study of history. . . . By working with these rhythms, we can protect our health, improve our professional productivity and better understand both ourselves and others.[4]

Chronobiologists have confirmed the existence of internal biological rhythms that operate automatically without our having to think about them. A decade ago there were over a hundred such rhythms identified and, no doubt, many more are categorized each year. These internal rhythms are broadly classified into three distinct groups according to the length of time between oscillations:

• Ultradian—cycles less than a day long (examples: heartbeat, breathing, digestion, brain waves);

- Circadian—cycles about a day long (examples: sleep/wake, body temperature, heart rate); and
- Infradian—cycles greater than a day long (examples: women's menstrual cycles, reproduction, seasonal immunity).

A common thread to several internal body rhythms is the impact of light. From the Scriptures' "Let there be light," to the Aztecs worshiping the sun god, light has held a sacred fascination from the dawn of civilization. In current times, scientists have been studying light in a desanctified manner in a quest to better understand its mysterious properties. Albert Einstein said he'd spent fifty years brooding over a specific question about light and was no closer to an answer than when he started. Forty years after Einstein's death, physicist Arthur Zajonc noted, "Efforts to understand light have not abated. . . . The essence of light remains an enigma."[5] Einstein also once stated, "Light is the shadow of God."[6] It appears there's no escaping the draw of spirituality and mysticism when it comes to light energy.*

Regardless of exactly what light is, we do know that many circadian rhythms are diurnal, meaning they cycle in tune with day and night. Light waves—perhaps the ultimate rhythm—oscillate to various frequencies and enter our eyes, the windows of the soul. Once we receive the light waves, a multitude of remarkable internal processes regulate our many body cycles. As Jacob Liberman, therapist, educator, and author of *Light: Medicine of the Future*, puts it, "The sun, acting as our solar system's major conductor, truly keeps our internal orchestra functioning in harmony."[7]

VISION RHYTHMS

Before I get to Bates's primary discovery, let's consider a few common and well-known vision rhythms. You're already ahead of me if you

---

*For a fascinating discussion on the history of light, from the spiritual to the scientific, refer to Zajonc's masterpiece, *Catching the Light: The Entwined History of Light and Mind*.

immediately thought of blinking, an ultradian rhythm. When something happens "in the blink of an eye," it is indeed fairly fast; the eyelids close in about a quarter to half a second. The average frequency, or rate, of blinking seems to be in the range of once every two to four seconds. Although blinking is an involuntary reflex, its speed and rate can be increased or decreased by a number of factors such as conscious control, fatigue, or anxiety.

Another commonly known eye rhythm is dilation and contraction of our pupils under changing light conditions. From dark to light, it takes about one minute for the eye pupil to contract from 8 mm to 3 mm, whereas from light to dark, it takes about six minutes to dilate from 3 mm to 8 mm. This rhythm depends mostly on environmental factors for its frequency. Theoretically, if a person were exposed to constant illumination for an entire day, the pupil size would remain stable and would change only at night. In reality, however, people are exposed to constantly changing light conditions throughout the day; some changes may be sudden, but most are gradual.

No doubt, you've experienced this next rhythm firsthand yourself many times when entering a darkened room (such as a movie theater) after being outside in the bright sunshine. The sudden change is literally blinding, as you cannot seem to see much of anything right away. Vision science has measured this rhythmic adaptation from lightness to darkness and vice versa. Going from bright surroundings to a darkened room is a slow process. It takes between fifteen to twenty-five minutes for your eyes to adjust to 80 percent of their night vision and an hour to fully adjust. The reverse, adapting to lightness from darkness, is blazing fast in comparison. It's a two-phase process, where the first phase is about 0.05 second for the eyes to become half adjusted. The second phase occurs more gradually to adapt the remaining 50 percent of your day vision.

Other eye rhythms are so fast that blinking is an absolute slowpoke in comparison. When you gaze at an object and focus your attention on it, your eyes aren't like a camera on a tripod at that point. A veritable microscopic symphony is playing continuously with tiny rhythmic movements including flicks (also called microsaccades), drifts, and tremors. Tremors, as the name implies, are high-frequency vibrations that constantly micro-oscillate the eyeball to keep the central portion stimulated with light rays from the image being viewed. These tremors cycle at thirty to seventy times per second, as fast as the vibration produced by a string played on a bass guitar. If your center of focus drifts ever so slightly off the object, then a flick—a jumping motion—occurs to reposition the image.

The orchestra of microrhythms and other eye motions plays on through the night. Studying the cycles of rapid eye movement (REM) during sleep has been a significant aspect of chronobiology research. When we dream, we are in a phase of REM sleep, and our eyes literally see it all as they dart from side to side, up, down, and around. Even the eye-blink reflex continues during sleep. Non-REM sleep is both a transition phase and deep-sleep phase when we aren't dreaming. Non-REM and REM sleep phases alternate every ninety minutes throughout the night. Interestingly, the REM cycle gets longer with each successive phase—from about five minutes in the first REM phase during the wee hours, to as long as an hour in the last cycle before awakening. Although the chronobiologists have tracked and recorded REM sleep in great detail, why it cycles in ninety-minute phases is still a grand mystery.

Chronobiologists recently discovered another rhythmic aspect to the eyes, using specially bred blind mice. Even though the mice had no image photoreceptors in their eyes to see, the mice retained the ability to regulate their circadian rhythms. According to Russell Foster, the head researcher, he "first found data in 1991 that indicated the eyes had a light-detecting system connected to the internal body clock," in addition to the previously known vision-producing light receptors. He ran into the proverbial brick wall of total skepticism. He said he "had real problems publishing it at that time. The attitude (from other scientists) was that the eye has been studied for 150 years and you can't possibly tell them that there's another light detecting system there."[8] It seems Foster had only a taste of what Bates dealt with his entire career and what natural-vision specialists currently continue to face from the orthodoxy.

TO AND FRO

In the introduction, I mentioned that I began the Bates Method of NVI with only a scant understanding from an indirect source of some of Bates's teachings. Before starting I was confident the method would work for me. I also made the assumption that the improvement would be linear, gradually getting better each day, month, and year until one day I would maybe achieve 20/20 vision. What happened within a few weeks of undertaking NVI completely threw that assumption out the window.

As I described, one afternoon while walking home from the office with my glasses in my pocket, I had a brief glimpse of near-perfect vision for a few seconds. The experience totally stunned and shocked me. The clarity just came out of the blue without my trying to do anything. I could distinctly see the shape of a stop sign about three blocks ahead. As quickly as the clear sight came, it faded back to blur. You can imagine my elation as I rushed home to tell my family.

In the next few weeks, I began to have more of these glimpses of near-perfect sight outside from time to time and eventually started to have them inside under artificial light as well. The strange thing was, if I tried to *make* them happen, they wouldn't. I eventually got used to the brief episodes of clear sight coming and going on their own when I wasn't expecting them.

Another observation about my natural vision also confused me once I could do most office work without wearing glasses. I found that my vision under steady artificial light conditions would be reasonably clear during the morning for computer-monitor work and close-up deskwork. If I then went outside during the noon hour, I would see better because of the greater intensity of the light from the bright sunshine. The sharper vision was also a result of my pupils contracting to a very small diameter, causing less scattering of the peripheral light rays in the eyes—what vision science calls the "pinhole effect." (The effect permits light rays to fall most efficiently on the retina's central zone of clearest perception.) However, when I returned to the office after lunch, my indoor vision would be considerably worse than it had been during the morning. There was an initial period of lighter-to-darker adjustment, but the visual blur would last the whole afternoon, and my vision never really came back to the same level of clarity as in the morning. As well as confusing, it was also very annoying.

From both these observations of my own vision, it became apparent that NVI was anything but linear. My sight seemed to be improving in waves. It certainly left me pondering. How could my daytime vision without glasses go from very blurry to almost 20/20 in an instant so soon into my vision-improvement program? And why was this improvement of such short duration? What was causing my eyesight to worsen after exposure to bright light, and why would it take so long to become clearer again? Little did I realize it at the time, but Dr. Bates had studied and documented these very phenomena over eighty years before and, through tireless and relentless research and analysis, found out why they occurred.

CONVENTIONAL EYE MODEL

Orthodox medicine treats humans as machines with various parts, such as a structural frame (skeleton), a protective coating (skin), elastomeric fibers (muscles), a pump (heart), a bellows (lungs), plumbing (veins and arteries), a computer (brain), and, of course, cameras (eyes) to see the world. Modeling humans in this fashion is also referred to as reductionism; the whole is divided into many individual parts, and although connected, they are presumed to be independent in function. The lines and divisions go from the visible outer all the way to the inner submicroscopic level. Taoism says we should know when to quit this endless division:

> *Once the whole is divided, the parts need names.*
> *There are already enough names.*
> *One must know when to stop.*[9]

The mechanical modeling of the eye can be traced to the era of Hermann von Helmholtz, a renowned German scientist and ophthalmologist. As part of his research, he theorized that the crystalline lens inside our eyes is the sole mechanism of what's called *accommodation*—the ability of the eye to change focus from near to far and vice versa. That theory was on somewhat shaky ground from the beginning, not being overwhelmingly conclusive, yet it quickly became dogma. A hundred and fifty or so years later, heated debates still rage in vision science as to what mechanical part, or parts, of the eye make it change focus.

There's no doubting that Helmholtz was a brilliant medical researcher, but consider for a moment his bias, and that of the entire era. He was one of four German scientists who "swore a celebrated oath to account for all processes of the body in purely physiochemical terms. . . . It was in direct conflict with a style of medicine that had existed for centuries, if not millennia—a medicine which believed that the patient's inner life and social being" were absolutely vital in the healing process.[10] Helmholtz had confidently stated, "The object of the natural sciences is to find the motions upon which all other changes are based, and their corresponding motive forces—to resolve themselves, therefore, into *mechanics* [emphasis added]." He had even "once made disparaging remarks about the human eye and suggested specific mechanical improvements."[11]

Once the eye had been modeled as a machine, a means to measure vision was needed. One method developed was an eye chart that people would read to determine their visual acuity relative to a quantitative normal standard. The normal standard that was set for good vision was 20/20. The eye chart method is referred to as a "subjective" test, as an eye care professional simply relies on the subject's personal responses to determine the result.

Another method of measurement developed was a so-called "objective" test, since the subject being tested provided no direct feedback This method involved an eye specialist shining a light inside a person's eye to gauge the refractive state. *Refraction* is a technical term that denotes the bending of light rays through a medium such as glass or water. A very common example of refraction is when you place a spoon in a glass of water. The metal appears distorted at the water surface due to the light refraction.

Refraction also occurs when light enters our eyes. The light rays must pass through both some liquid and the lens inside each eye. If a person has normal vision, there is said to be no refractive error. The light rays bend and converge in such a way as to create a clear image on the light receptors in the back of the eye (the retina). If a person has blurry vision, then a measurable error of refraction is said to occur because the light rays aren't converging properly on the retina.

Bates's formal medical training had taught him the mechanical-eye theory, which suggested that a normal eye with clear vision was like a perfect machine, always in good working order. Furthermore, the theory went on to suggest that abnormal vision (a refractive error) was a continuous condition due to a permanently deformed eyeball. Theory is one thing; experience is quite another.

REFRACTIVE RHYTHM

During his many years of clinical practice and research, Bates couldn't help but observe numerous cases of anomalies to the conventional eye theory. "Examining 30,000 pairs of eyes a year at the New York Eye and Ear Infirmary and other institutions," he wrote, "I observed many cases in which errors of refraction either recovered spontaneously, or changed their form, and I was unable either to ignore them, or to satisfy myself with the orthodox explanations, even where such explanations were available. It seemed to me that if a [theory] is a truth it must always be a truth. There can be no exceptions."[12] He came to the conclusion that he would have march to an entirely different beat if he was to understand what he kept observing time and time again. After years of exhaustive experimentation he stated, "I discovered many facts which had not previously been known, and which I was quite unable to reconcile with the orthodox teachings on the subject. . . . [This] left me no choice but to reject the entire body of orthodox teaching about . . . errors of refraction."[13]

What Bates initially thought to be an exception to a rule turned out to be the perfectly natural way the eye functions. Rather than a refractive state being fixed and permanent as the orthodox theory suggested, eye refraction is flexible and changing under many circumstances and conditions. In essence, eyesight is a rhythm that is in continual flux. Bates described the ebb and flow of vision further:

> During thirty years devoted to the study of refraction, I have found few people who could maintain perfect sight for more than a few minutes at a time, even under the most favorable conditions; and often I have seen the refraction change half a dozen times or more in a second, the variations ranging all the way from twenty diopters of myopia [severe nearsightedness] to normal. Similarly I have found no eyes with continuous or unchanging errors of refraction, all persons with errors of refraction having, at frequent intervals during the day and night, moments of normal vision, when their myopia, hypermetropia [farsightedness], or astigmatism [the eyeball is out-of-round] wholly disappears. The form of the error also changes, myopia even changing into hypermetropia, and one form of astigmatism into another.[14]

The discovery of this refractive rhythm was the basis for developing his entire method of improving sight by natural means. It is what I consider to be Bates's first core fact in NVI:

> No refractive state, whether it is normal or abnormal, can be permanent.[15]

Throughout his career, Bates examined the eyes of "tens of thousands of school children, hundreds of infants and thousands of animals." He checked the refractive state of subjects under numerous conditions, such as:

- At rest and in motion (and sometimes when Bates himself was moving);
- Asleep and awake;

- Under the influence of ether and chloroform;
- Eye pupils contracted in the daytime and dilated at night;
- Comfortable and excited;
- Trying hard to see and relaxing to see;
- Lying and telling the truth;
- Squinting and not squinting; and
- Oscillating the eyes from side to side, up and down, and in other directions.

What he observed and documented from these various circumstances can be categorized as follows:

School Children

Of the twenty thousand school children Bates examined in one year, more than half had normal eyesight. Yet none had perfect sight in each eye continually throughout the day. Bates found their sight "might be good in the morning and imperfect in the afternoon, or imperfect in the morning and perfect in the afternoon." Many children could read one type of vision test chart with excellent sight but were unable to read a different chart with the same degree of clarity. Several children "could also read some letters of the alphabet perfectly, while unable to distinguish other letters of the same size under similar conditions. The degree of this imperfect sight varied within wide limits, from one-third to one-tenth, or less. Its duration was also variable."[16]

Discomfort

Mental discomfort such as depression, anger, or anxiety always produced blur in normal eyes and increased the degree of blur for someone with imperfect sight. People subjected to physical discomfort, such as pain, cough, fever, or extreme heat or cold, would similarly experience a lowering of vision. NVI therapist Janet Goodrich states, "During illness, negative emotional states, and fatigue, the visual energy may abate and perception diminish for a time. But it is never lost."[17]

Strong Light

This is the condition I described earlier that affected my improving vision. I remember being extremely sensitive to bright sunshine as a child. As an adult, I also wore *photochromic* lenses for several years (in aviator frames, for a stylish, "cool" appearance), which automatically darkened outside and lightened indoors, further reducing my tolerance and natural adjustment to bright light. Bates found that a "sudden exposure to strong light, or rapid or sudden changes of light, are likely to produce imperfect sight in the normal eye, continuing in some cases for weeks and months."[18] He further found this impact more pronounced in people with imperfect sight because of a sluggish or impaired dark-to-light pupil response. He also found that those with imperfect sight were usually affected even more by exposure to bright light than people with normal vision.

Sleep

I'm assuming Bates had some subjects who were very deep sleepers, so he could open their eyelids to check the refractive state of their eyes without disturbing them. Some people who had normal vision when awake would exhibit various types of refractive errors when they were asleep. Those with imperfect sight increased their refractive error during sleep. Bates concluded, "This is why people waken in the morning with eyes more tired than at any other time, or even [waken] with severe headaches."[19] He observed similar findings when people were anaesthetized under ether or chloroform, or unconscious from some other cause.

Miscellaneous

When people looked at an unfamiliar object, their vision lowered due to an error of refraction.

When people were subjected to an unexpected loud noise, they all experienced a lowering of vision. (Several years later, Russian researchers verified that loud city noises narrowed the field of vision for many people.[20])

Infants' eyes were also checked, and their refractive state was found to be continually changing. Children produced an error of refraction when they told an obvious lie.

Bates used an instrument called a *retinoscope* to shine a highly focused light inside a person's eye. The refractive rhythm could be detected by observing changes in the retinal reflex (the reflection of light coming from the back of the eye). The retinoscope is a staple of the eye-care profession to this day, and other professionals have found that refraction is not an unwavering condition.

Many years after Bates made these observations, other researchers have verified the refractive rhythm of the eyes. Raymond Gottlieb, a behavioral optometrist who improved his myopia by practicing the Bates Method, reported the findings of Gesell and colleagues. They observed changes in refraction of children who were performing various tasks and noted that the "variations . . . are not random . . . [but] a two-way, reciprocating process—a directional process which emanates from within the self, goes out, and then returns within."[21] The researchers discovered these "two distinguishable phases" when a child first looked at the examiner's face and then looked at and touched an interesting toy. The child's refractive state would be slightly myopic (nearsighted) in the first case and then slightly hyperopic (farsighted) in the second instance.

In his practice of optometry, Roberto Kaplan observed that changes in the retinal reflex depended on the person's participation in the eye-testing process. If someone visualized events or thought of episodes that conjured different emotions, the reflex changed markedly. "I could see," he wrote, "that the person's thoughts and feelings were influencing the light presence in his or her eyes."[22]

Otis Brown, an aeronautical engineer who has helped numerous pilots reverse their myopia and improve their vision, has scientifically studied refraction of the eye. He concludes that the "experimental facts demonstrate that all eyes change their focal state as the visual environment is changed." The eye is never locked in one refractive position like the old-time "box cameras" but is more like an autofocusing system.[23]

Similarly, Merrill Bowan, a neurodevelopmental optometrist, describes recent evidence in vision science that suggests the manner in which our eyes focus "functions primarily as an oscillating analyzer with a dual-phase mechanism."[24] In other words, when we look at an object, its image on the retina oscillates rapidly to and fro until the eyes bring it in most clearly in our central vision.

Armed with the information Bates had presented, the brief glimpses of near-perfect vision I was experiencing from time to time early in my vision-improvement process now made sense. The natural refractive rhythm of my eyes was starting to come back slowly but surely. It had been forced into, and stuck, in one artificial refractive state for years behind rigid prescription lenses. The returning range of the fluctuation from blur to clarity and back again was quite dramatic, but the phenomenon is nothing spectacular. It is a routine aspect of NVI, which Bates called a *flash*.

THE FLASH

Many people who begin undertaking NVI experience brief periods of near-perfect sight while not wearing glasses or contact lenses. Because these "flashes" come without warning, they can be emotionally overwhelming. I've personally been overcome with tears and overjoyed by euphoria all at once. Others have been similarly affected.

Soo Tan, an Australian optometrist, partook in a vision-improvement seminar conducted by Jacob Liberman in 1993. The seminar was specifically conducted for progressively minded optometrists wanting to gain firsthand experience of NVI. What they were learning contradicted everything they were taught in their formal vision education. Soo's vision improvement during the course of a weekend was the most dramatic. Without glasses, her acuity tested 20/600 at the start of the seminar, a highly myopic condition. She then learned some simple concepts that allowed her refractive rhythm to reawaken, all the while without wearing glasses. Six hours later her vision tested 20/225, almost a threefold improvement in that short time frame. But most amazing, twenty-four hours after the start of the seminar, her unaided vision for a brief moment tested virtually 20/25 (she had only three errors on the line)! In her own words, "The numbers seemed to be doubled and blurry one moment and then suddenly clear the next. It was unbelievable! I was so shocked that I cried for ten minutes."[25]

Other people have experienced a similar temporary improvement in their vision after removing their glasses for a time to unleash the suspended refractive rhythm. Its impact can be equally profound; for Tom Quackenbush, it was a life-altering encounter. He had severe nearsightedness, with a resultant visual acuity of 20/800. In his words, "I experienced a dramatic improvement in my eyesight for approximately one hour while participating in a stress reduction program; this occurred *before* I knew about the Bates method."[26] After discovering the Bates Method and NVI, Quackenbush eventually abandoned his career as an analytical chemist to become a certified NVI instructor, a trainer of other certified instructors, and an author.

There's no disputing the flash. It wasn't something that Bates made up or embellished. The phenomenon has been well documented and experienced by many other people in subsequent generations. The numerous students who have studied and practiced the modern-day Bates Method and/or NVI training have reported flashes of improved eyesight. The optometrists who formed the American Vision Institute (the AVI offers a therapeutic vision-improvement program different from the Bates Method) write that "*clear flashes* . . . are periods of clear vision without 'corrective' lenses. These are quite common and have even been reported by people with really poor vision. With perseverance, the clear flashes usually become longer and more intense."[27]

EYESTRAIN

When professional golfers compete under intense pressure during an important event, one of the first things to go wrong in their swings is their rhythm. The surge of bodily changes suddenly becomes very problematic, and they have great difficulty finding the regular tempo and feel they normally have under less-stressful situations. The over-all rhythm is affected because so many of the body rhythms drastically change, especially the heartbeat and respiration rate. Because these rhythms speed up, the tendency is for movement and tempo to speed up as well. Any type of fine activity that requires rhythm and grace is difficult to control under emotional stress. Imagine what happens to the body rhythms under more continual stress.

Chronobiologists have studied these changes and have found that our body cycles go somewhat berserk under prolonged stress. The most noticeable change is that our days begin to lengthen. The circadian cycles may extend two or more hours. The extra energy during the day is a tradeoff, for at night, a person gets less sleep. It may eventually lead to insomnia. Other shorter cycles may become desynchronized; body temperature changes may fall out of sync with sleep/wake cycles; when it's dinner time, the digestive system may be in a holding pattern; or we're keyed up for demanding tasks when we should be slowing down. A case of the blues may end up becoming full-blown depression. The body cycles go even more awry under this severe mental condition.

For vision cycles, emotional strain similar to that produced by fear or anger causes the pupils to dilate. The blink rate also becomes much faster, and eye movements become jerky and helter-skelter in the attempt to see as much as possible quickly. Long before the negative conse-quences of stress and strain to our health were recognized and widely accepted, Bates observed another adverse effect on eyesight. The large fluctuations in refractive rhythm he observed were the direct result of a strain to see:

> The eye with normal sight never tries to see. If for any reason, such as the dimness of the light, or the distance of the object, it cannot see a particular point, it shifts to another. It never tries to bring out the point by staring at it, as the eye with imperfect sight is con-stantly doing. . . . The act of seeing is passive. Things are seen, just as they are felt, or heard, or tasted, without effort or volition on the part of the subject. When sight is perfect the letters on the test card

are waiting, perfectly black and perfectly distinct, to be recognized. They do not have to be sought; they are there. In imperfect sight they are sought and chased. The eye goes after them. An effort is made to see them.[28]

Bates noted that people with good vision had eye movements that were "short, rhythmical and easy," whereas people with imperfect sight had movements that were "longer, irregular and accompanied by strain."[29] He further noted that, if the strain became more continuous, a person's eyesight would "steadily deteriorate and may eventually be destroyed."[30] His observations about the impact of mental strain are what I consider to be the second core fact in his teachings.

> Mental strain of any kind always produces a conscious or unconscious eyestrain and if the strain takes the form of an effort to see, an error of refraction is always produced.[31]

As Bates pointed out, the source of this strain came from within civilized society itself. "Visual acuity," he wrote, "declines as civilization advances. Under the conditions of civilized life men's minds are under a continual strain. They have more things to worry them than uncivilized man had, and they are not obliged to keep cool and collected in order that they may see and do other things upon which existence depends. If he allowed himself to get nervous, primitive man was promptly eliminated; but civilized man survives and transmits his mental characteristics to posterity."[32]

Recent research affirms exactly what Bates had steadfastly maintained. A study of vision-science literature over several generations reveals that there have been at least nineteen theories developed on the cause of blurred vision, particularly nearsightedness. Because some of these theories were related, Merrill Bowan was able to consolidate the list to seven. Although no one theory stands out as the definitive culprit, a common link does exist, and the list was further pared down: "All seven . . . reduce to one: Stress . . . in the form of any imposed stimulation, appears to be the unifying element in all refractive error and personality style appears to be the dependent variable modifying the error."[33]

The degree of mental strain, then, depends on how the *beholder* responds to the stresses of modern living, as noted by behavioral optometrist Richard Kavner: "Vision is tied up with how a person moves, thinks, comes to a decision; visual problems can give us clues to what kinds of stresses the person operates under. Distortions of the eye are considered to be problems in reaching a decision, reflections of behavioral style, and indications of some form of stress, whether it be physiological, cultural or environmental."[34]

For civilization to prosper, children need to be fully educated to serve important roles. Unfortunately, that's when most vision problems begin to develop and multiply.

STRAIN IN SCHOOL

Ultimately, indoctrination in the rat race begins very early in life. Although the written agenda of schooling is supposedly a formal education, the unwritten agenda is a different type of training. Students quickly learn all sorts of rules they must follow, particularly punctuality to the clock and bells, adherence to a proper dress code, talking only at designated times, and above all, obeying (fearing) authority.

In Bates's day, and even when I was a child, the use of strict discipline and corporal punishment was a standard part of teaching. As he said, "The various fear incentives still so largely employed by teachers . . . have the effect, usually, of completely paralyzing minds already benumbed by lack of interest, and the effect upon the vision is equally disastrous."[35] Although the physical abuse of children in the name of discipline is no longer tolerated, the specter of fear prevails to this day. Children figure out quickly that conformity to the system is the supreme good; individuality labels you as a troublemaker. As for the education itself, children understand that getting good grades is the name of the game. Bates commented further:

In the process of education civilized children are shut up for hours every day within four walls, in the charge of teachers who are too often nervous and irritable. [The children] are even compelled to remain for long periods in the same position. The things they are required to learn may be presented in such a way as to be excessively uninteresting; and they are under a continual compulsion to think of the gaining of marks and prizes rather than the acquisition of knowledge for its own sake. Some children endure these unnatural conditions better than others. Many cannot stand the strain, and thus the schools become the hotbed, not only of myopia, but of all other errors of refraction.[36]

Based on recent vision research, Merrill Bowan has concluded that the classroom is a "breeding ground" for the onset of blurred vision. "A child in a desk for hours each school day," he wrote, "is in an artificial environment highly unlike the natural environment for which the human body was designed. . . . Children's actual responses to school desk containment will vary, of course, [but the] school desk and its reduction of the opportunities for movement is a similar environment to that of the laboratory animal."[37] Simply being confined like a caged animal is one stressor that leads to mental strain and eyestrain.

Other stressors in the classroom include performance, situational, and social anxiety. Students spend countless extra hours doing homework, and a great deal of effort is required to memorize information to be regurgitated for tests, only to forget it all a few days later. Bates commented further on this very obsession with forced memorization in the schools:

This idea [of effort] is drilled into us from our cradles. The whole educational system is based upon it; and in spite of the wonderful results attained by Montessori through the total elimination of every species of compulsion in the educational process, educators who call themselves modern still cling to the club, under various disguises, as a necessary auxiliary to the process of imparting knowledge. . . .

Under the present educational system there is a constant effort to compel the children to remember. These efforts always fail. They spoil both the memory and the sight. The memory cannot be forced any more than the vision can be forced.[38]

Sadly, this type of compulsion in the educational system is taken to extremes in the Eastern countries nowadays, in their desperate race to become more modernized and highly competitive economically. As observed by Alan MacFarlane and Gerry Martin, authors and historians specializing in the history of glass, schoolchildren there can spend extraordinary hours doing schoolwork in and out of the classroom:

We summarize a visit to a Korean girls' middle school as follows: "Visit girls' middle school and are allowed to film a class learning Korean. . . . Children start school at 8.30 a.m., finish at 4.30 p.m., then go to 'crammers' where, in bad light and general noise, they continue to study until 10 p.m. We were told that when they return home they often engage in Internet chat until 2 a.m. Their eyes have about five hours' rest." By the age of seventeen, they might well have extended the cramming period to beyond midnight. There are very few breaks for games, cultural activities or anything else.[39]

The pressures and demands in Japanese culture have been well documented by Westerners, who once envied Japan's industrial prowess before its markets came crashing down. The Japanese obsession with the work ethic is considered the pinnacle of duty and sacrifice. What we don't appreciate is just how early this particular attitude is fostered in children. "In Japan . . . children often go to pre-school and start serious education when they are three or four. . . . Big department stores have areas which specialize in recommending and selling the appropriate clothes for mothers who are taking their tiny infants for an interview at a good kindergarten." And there is "the famous image of Japanese children sitting past midnight in the cramming establishments, literally holding their eyelids open with matchsticks."[40]

Whether the tasks in and out of school call for effort, striving, competition, fear, or exhaustion, the net result is the same for many children—mental strain and eyestrain. The visual difficulties that arise from the constant eyestrain have resulted in a massive problem in society, one of epidemic proportions.

STARING

Have you ever played the card game Concentration, also called Memory? If you haven't, the game starts out with two people placing a deck of cards face down in neat rows and columns. The first player randomly selects two cards and turns them face up. If the two cards are a matching pair, such as kings, then that player wins those cards and removes them from play. If the two cards turned up are not a matching pair, they are placed back face down and kept in play. The next player randomly picks another two cards. If the first card turned over is a six, and the player remembers that the opponent turned up a six on the previous turn, the player has to remember exactly where that initial six is situated in the rows and columns. If the player remembers correctly and turns over the first six, then the second player keeps that pair. The goal of the game is to win more matching pairs than your opponent.

My wife and I taught our kids this game for fun when they were preschoolers. Who do you think won the most? It certainly wasn't Mom or Dad, university-educated adults with lots of experience. At their tender young age, our kids absolutely annihilated us at this card game. I can recall some games where I would win only three or four pairs! I just couldn't believe how good the kids' memories were. When they saw a card turned up that was a match to a previously turned-up card, they knew just where to go to make a match! It was almost as if they had X-ray vision. I, on the other hand, would struggle trying to remember where I saw a specific card turned up before, and I would have to guess. Most times I would be wrong.

My many years of formal education had focused heavily on concentration, the very name of the game, but it didn't seem to help in this situation. It seemed the more I tried to concentrate on remembering specific card locations the more it backfired. Our kids weren't yet indoctrinated with "education" and the supposed importance of knowing how to concentrate hard, so their ability to recall vividly came naturally and spontaneously.

My concentration skills were further put to the test beyond the classroom. As a boy, I took many years of formal piano lessons and music theory (the Royal Conservatory method) and the emphasis was rote learning, heavy on structure, notation, keys, scales, proper hand and wrist position, and so forth. I would spend hours practicing, straining my eyes through strong glasses to read the sheet music while simultaneously playing the piano. Perfectionism was drilled into me—practice makes perfect. I felt that I wasn't supposed to make mistakes, and the more I concentrated on avoiding them, the more pressure would build. Each time I replayed a certain song and got closer to a part I'd botched before, I'd get anxious. This anxiety would expand like air in a balloon. I hoped to sail through the troublesome section without a problem, and maybe I would. But then, bang went the anxiety balloon—I'd eventually make a mistake somewhere else. Arrgghh!

To play a song from start to finish without any mistakes *exactly* the way it was written out seemed to be the whole goal of learning the piano. It wasn't about the joy of playing freely in your own style whatever you happened to enjoy, mistakes included. It was just so regimented, much like an assembly line. The styles of music I had to play seemed to be too complicated and were not what I enjoyed listening to. When it came time for recital competitions, the pressure was more intense; my nervousness would cause me to sweat and shake uncontrollably. It just wasn't much fun, so, like many kids, I gradually quit playing the piano.

Mental strain in formalized schooling and other types of structured training translates into much immobilization; creativity, imagination, memory, spontaneity all get stifled and, some may even suggest, "blocked" and "destroyed" during the process of rote learning.[41] Mental strain in the form of excessive concentration is equally as bad for the eyes, and Bates continually warned of the dangers:

The dictionary defines "Concentration" as an effort to see one thing only, or to do one thing only. I have never met any person who was able to concentrate on a point for any length of time. Concentration is impossible. Trying to do the impossible is a strain; which is the main cause of imperfect sight. For we find that all persons with imperfect sight try to concentrate—try to imagine things stationary. . . . To stare, strain or try to concentrate is an effort which is followed by not only imperfect sight, but symptoms of discomfort, pain and fatigue.[42]

The idea that the attention can be forced is a very common one and is very bad for the eyes. It is greatly encouraged by popular writers, but contrary to the teachings of more reliable psychologists, who know that forced attention can only be momentary, and that it is a great strain upon the mind and the whole body.[43]

Rapt attention does not mean "wrapped" attention, where your mind is tied up under lock and key on the subject matter before you. When you're driving a car along a busy stretch of highway, you definitely want to be attentive to the task. Multitasking may be a desirable trait in certain jobs, but it has proven to be deadly behind the wheel. Many fatal crashes are caused by drivers diverting their attention from the road to fidgeting with radio dials or talking on cell phones. That's why many jurisdictions have banned the use of cell phones when driving a vehicle. On one hand, being actively attentive to constantly changing stimuli does not imply forced concentration. On the other hand, driving a monotonous stretch of highway at night with no other traffic can be quite a strain on the eyes and can be very tiring. Is this perhaps an example of forced concentration? How many people have fallen asleep while driving under such unchanging stimuli? So attentiveness is being mindful of what's before your eyes, but not being forced to pay close attention for a prolonged period without some sort of change. William James, one of the "reliable psychologists" of Bates's era, spoke of this sort of attentiveness as a "beat" or "pulse":

One often hears it said that genius is nothing but a power of sustained attention, and the popular impression probably prevails that men of genius are remarkable for their voluntary powers in this direction. *But a little introspective observation will show any one that voluntary attention cannot be continuously sustained— that it comes in beats.* When we are studying an uninteresting subject, if our mind tends to wander, we have to bring back our attention every now and then by using distinct pulses of effort, which revivify the topic for a moment, the mind then running on for a certain number of seconds or minutes with spontaneous interest, until again some intercurrent idea captures it and takes it off. Then the processes of volitional recall must be repeated once more. Voluntary attention, in short, is only a momentary affair. . . . Try to attend steadfastly to a dot on the paper or on the wall. You presently find that one or the other of two things has happened: either your field of vision has become blurred, so that you now see nothing distinct at all, or else you have involuntarily ceased to look at the dot in question, and are looking at something else. But, if you ask yourself successive questions about the dot—how big it is, how far, of what shape, what shade of color, etc.; in other words, if you turn it over, if you think of it in various ways, and along with various kinds of associates—you can keep your mind on it for a comparatively long time.[44]

Bates had said that you could have good vision when looking at the stars in the night sky, but if you tried to count all the stars in a particular constellation, you would likely have an error of refraction, becoming temporarily nearsighted. Whenever Bates's patients tried to look at one letter on an eye chart for too long or tried to see all letters equally clearly, the letters would become blurry, and the person would feel discomfort. In one case, a person was able to see the letter *K* on the eye chart with clear vision, but when he was asked to count all the corners in the *K*, the letter fuzzed out on him.

These types of efforts to concentrate are cognitive tasks such as categorizing and reasoning. As behavioral optometrist Raymond Gottlieb notes, the categorizing task could be thought of as, "What is it?" and the reasoning task, "What is to be done?" He suggests that a rabbit caught between two aggressive dogs, one to the left and one to the right, would be initially immobilized. The rabbit would be highly keyed up with anxiety, knowing the "what is it," but then would have to *concentrate* on "what is to be done" before taking action. For children in a classroom setting, the categorizing and reasoning is not under such threatening situations but is continual and "dogged" throughout each day. This cognitive strain causes muscle tension, most notably in the eyebrows, and, Gottlieb says, "Optometrists are aware of changes in the eyeball during reasoning tasks such as math problems."[45] As Huxley pointed out, "The power of seeing is greatly lowered by distressing emotional states," and conscious effort "can interfere with the processes of seeing even at times when no distressing emotions are present." It's because mental interference, such as "trying too hard to do well, or . . . feeling unduly anxious about possible mistakes," causes strain.[46]

Think of proper vision, then, as being as vital as breathing. If you were to hold your breath for too long, the strain and tension would build to such a point that you might pass out. If you "hold your mind" to concentrate or stare, the strain causes your vision to "pass out," in a sense. You mustn't interfere with the natural pulse and beat of your eyesight. By all means be attentive, but avoid staring. Maintain your refractive rhythm to be in tune with the Tao.

JUST THE FACTS

Much like the *Dragnet* homicide detective asking questions of a witness, Bates was interested in just the facts. He preferred facts to theories because he was immersed in the common-sense world of day-to-day reality in his profession. He practiced the time-honored tradition of *empiricism*—finding valuable facts and discoveries through observation and experiment in the absence of any theory. Theoretical science concerns itself with simple systems, whereas empirical research like

Bates's is suited to complex systems under diverse conditions.*

As discussed already, Bates found far too many facts that were glaring exceptions to the long-held mechanistic theory of how the human eye supposedly focused. He stated, "In the science of ophthalmology, theories, often stated as facts, have served to obscure the truth and throttle investigation for more than a hundred years. The explanations . . . have caused us to ignore or explain away a multitude of facts which otherwise would have led to the discovery of the truth about errors of refraction and the consequent prevention of an incalculable amount of human misery."[47] The theories were far too simple for such a complex system as the human eye.

Because he eventually concluded he had no choice but to reject the orthodox teachings, Bates felt compelled to offer his own explanation of what accounted for the changing refractive states he observed. "Instead of starting out with a working hypothesis," he wrote, "it is my custom to accumulate as many facts as I possibly can, to analyze these facts in various ways and by every method known to science to try to discover whether my facts are true or not; and, believe me, that is not always an easy thing to do."[48] He toiled tirelessly for years on his own time and at his own expense before he was satisfied that he had a reasonable physiological explanation of how the eye focused. But when presenting his findings, he was very careful to point out that he aimed to provide "a collection of facts and not of theories. . . . When explanations have been offered it has been done with considerable trepidation, because I have never been able to formulate a theory that would withstand the test of the facts either in my possession at the time, or accumulated later."[49] A man of integrity, he did not "fear successful contradiction" and openly encouraged professional colleagues throughout the country to find exceptions to any factual statements he made.

If you are interested in reading the in-depth technical details about the orthodox theory versus Bates's explanation, this information is doc-

---

*Chapter 8 explores the inherent flaws in the promulgation of theoretical science applied in practice.

umented both in *Relearning to See* and on the Web site www.iblindness
.org. But as Huxley stated, "Whether Dr. Bates was right or wrong in
his rejection of the Helmholtz theory . . . I am entirely unqualified to
say. . . . My concern is not with anatomical mechanism of accommodation, but with the art of seeing—and the art of seeing does not stand or
fall with any particular physiological hypothesis."[50]

I concur wholeheartedly. I'm not qualified to judge either, but Bates
must at least have been on a far better track than the old theory. Long
before I read about Bates's in-depth teachings, I was living and breathing several facts about my own vision every day, facts that turned out
to be in complete congruence with his discoveries. Sure, vision science
has done a great job at finding all sorts of "dots"—reducing the eye
to numerous parts to study their purpose and function. But the scientists haven't managed to connect the dots to explain how vision really
works in a unified way, nor have they unequivocally identified the cause
of blurred vision, let alone developed a cure for poor vision. A strictly
mechanical model of the eye can never be developed for something so
holistically complex as vision. Neurodevelopmental optometrist Merrill
Bowan recently stated, "It is futile, in the complexity of these [visual]
tasks, to artificially assign strictly unique functions to any single component part of the visual system. Each part appears to be involved in many
functions."[51]

While the establishment carefully guarded its majestic theory as an
immutable law for eternity, Bates meanwhile discovered two important facts: (1) refractive rhythm; and (2) the impact of mental strain on
vision. This in turn created tremendous hope. Conditions that for so
long had been thought of as irreversible and incurable could now possibly be improved or even fully cured. It became his life's work to find
ways to help people restore their eyesight by natural means. Bates was
especially dedicated in his concern for the welfare of children's vision,
working tirelessly to prevent and reverse the onslaught of myopia and a
lifetime dependence on artificial lenses.

4

SOFTNESS

All beings, grass and trees, when alive, are soft and bending,
When dead they are dry and brittle.
Therefore the hard and unyielding are companions of death,
The soft and yielding are companions of life.

Under heaven nothing is more soft and yielding than water.
Yet for attacking the solid and strong, nothing is better;
It has no equal.
The weak can overcome the strong;
The supple can overcome the stiff.

LAO TZU[1]

Bobby Jones was the Tiger Woods of his era. As the dominant competitive golfer in 1930, Jones won the Grand Slam of the time—the U.S. Amateur, U.S. Open, British Amateur, and British Open. To capture all four "majors" in a single season was a remarkable achievement, a feat many considered impossible. Walking along the fairway one day with sportswriter Grantland Rice, Jones began discussing the mystery of the golf swing. "I've discovered a man must play golf by 'feel,'" he said. "The hardest thing in the world to describe—but the easiest thing in the world to sense when you have it completely. . . . Today I have it completely. I don't have to think of anything . . . just meet the ball."[2]

In the current athletic vernacular, Jones was "in the zone" when he was playing golf that way. Obviously, we're not all born with the natural talent of a Jones or a Woods, but I'm sure we can all relate to the feeling of being in the zone in some activity or another. Whether it's in the performing arts, sports, school, or the business world, there are times when you can probably recall that feeling of effortless joy. You didn't have to force anything, and things went so well. If you could only bottle it up and repeat it at will!

We may not be born with star talents, but most of us are born with healthy eyes. As infants we instinctively used our eyes naturally, without conscious effort. If you're now hindered by visual blur, you've lost that innate ability and are straining to see. Softness is the key to clearing your vision as you embark on a journey to the effortless state of seeing naturally.

DYNAMIC WORLD

Physicist David Bohm once studied the inability of language to adequately describe various theories and findings in the emerging science of quantum physics. According to physicist and transpersonal psychologist Will Keepin, Bohm showed that the reliance on nouns in our modern languages imposes "strong, subtle pressures to see the world as fragmented and static. He emphasized that thought tends to create fixed structures in the mind, which can make dynamic entities seem to be static."[3] A case in point was my engineering education; the curriculum divided categories of *statics* and *dynamics* into separate classes devoted to the study of nonmoving and moving forces.

In contrast, ancient languages, such as Hebrew or those of the indigenous Native Americans, view the world as more process-oriented; everything is movement, flow, and transformation. These languages are more action oriented to match their worldview of flux. Physicist and psychology author F. David Peat, who collaborated with Bohm, explains, "Nouns as objects emerge in a secondary way through the modification of verbs. To them [the Blackfoot people of North America] the English language is a straight-jacket which forces their minds into a world of objects, categories and restrictive logic."[4]

A straightjacket is a good metaphor for the concentration and staring we discussed in the last chapter, severely restricting us during the reasoning and categorizing tasks we do each day. In reality, as the ancient civilizations are now showing us, *static* is purely an artificial designation. The world is in continuous flux, reaffirming the old adage, "The only constant is change." As Keepin puts it, when viewed in this context, "All objects are dynamic processes rather than static forms. To put it crudely, one could say that nouns do not really exist, only verbs exist. A noun is just a 'slow' verb; that is, it refers to a process that is progressing so slowly so as to appear static."[5]

Certain philosophers, mystics, and poets—seemingly disparate thinkers—agreed on this dynamic aspect of existence. Immanuel Kant, Jacob Boehme, and William Wordsworth saw everything as process and constant flow. The Greek philosopher Heraclitus viewed the world as a unified and orderly balance of dynamics. He was famous for stating, "Upon those who step into the same rivers different and ever different waters flow down." In other words, you never step in the same river twice. Plato understood this to mean that despite what our senses tell us, everything is always in flux.[6] Classifying the river as a thing implies an unchanging entity. The river appears static in that it is a distinct form on the landscape that is always there. But there is the ever-constant flow of water, the shifting contours of the riverbanks, the changing depths of the riverbed through scour and silting, and the rich and vast array of aquatic life that comes and goes. Individual appearances are static things we invent—the forms, shapes, and divisions we're so fond of sorting and categorizing.

"Nerves of steel" perhaps aren't so rock-solid after all. Even something as seemingly inert and permanent as steel changes shape and form in response to the environment. If you studied physics, you may have been taught that metals have a coefficient of expansion and contraction. If not, here's the translation: just like mercury—the silvery liquid metal in thermometers—steel expands in the heat and shrinks in the cold, and the amount of change is predictable and measurable. In our Canadian climate of extremes, a steel bridge girder 80 m (262 ft.) long is 77 mm (3 in.) shorter on the coldest day of winter than the hottest day of summer. Bridges are usually built with expansion joints to account for the movement. The other environmental dynamic property of steel results from exposure to water and air; unprotected steel corrodes (rusts) with time. The byproduct of rust is actually iron oxide, the very substance of the raw ore originally mined. Through intensely high-energy smelting and manufacturing processes, the iron is refined, mixed with a small amount of other elements such as carbon, and ultimately transformed into steel. But over a long period, the iron oxide simply returns to its natural state. Steel almost has a mind of its own! You never cross the same bridge twice.

Throughout the book, you'll note that from time to time I fall into the trap of static language. When discussing the negative effect of prescription glasses on our eyes, I use words like *immobilizing, rigid,* or *locked in.* Keep in mind that these terms are relative. Wearing glasses doesn't totally immobilize your eye movements. Glasses do, however, severely restrict the natural range of eye motions for normal functioning. The more powerful the lenses, the greater the impact on eye mobility. The net result is a hampered refractive rhythm.

Human activity is a continuum, where one end of the scale is minimal movement, and the other end, a great deal of movement. "Activity is a biological necessity," states Selye.[7] You simply cannot survive without movement. When we sleep, our muscles continue to move—only much less so than if we were awake and running a marathon—as we shift positions throughout the night. Our minds may be racing in sleep, however, with all sorts of wild dreams. There is also the continual motion of breathing, heartbeat, digestion, and the myriad other autonomic body functions. Regardless of which end of the activity spectrum we look at, healthy dynamics require minimal to no tension.

FLUID MOVEMENT

Taoists have a phrase, *wu wei,* that in English literally means "inaction" or "nonaction." Therein lies the fragmentary conundrum of our modern language. Huston Smith, author of *The World's Religions,* notes that such a translation suggests "a vacant attitude of idleness or abstention," a complete misinterpretation. To better capture the broader meaning of the phrase, he suggested "pure effectiveness" or "creative quietude":

> Creative quietude combines within a single individual two seemingly incompatible conditions—supreme activity and supreme relaxation. The seeming incompatibles can coexist because human beings are not self-enclosed entities. They ride an unbounded sea of *Tao* that sustains them, as we would say, through their subliminal minds. One way to create is through following the calculated directives of the conscious mind. The results of this mode of action, however, are seldom impressive; they tend to smack more of sorting and arranging than of inspiration. Genuine creation, as every artist knows, comes when the more abundant resources of the subliminal self are somehow tapped. But for this to happen a certain disassociation from the surface self is needed. The conscious mind must relax, stop standing in its own light, let go. Only so is it possible to break through the law of reversed effort in which the more we try the more our efforts boomerang.[8]

The "zone" in performing a skill could perhaps be substituted for wu wei. "A good athlete can enter a state of body-awareness in which the right stroke or the right movement happens by itself, effortlessly, without any interference of the conscious will," notes Stephen Mitchell in his translation of the Tao Te Ching. "This is a paradigm for nonaction: the purest and most effective form of action."[9] Musicians who improvise, or make up music as they go, rely on this effortless action to express themselves through their instruments. In their free-form performances, they commonly report feeling as though they're almost like a receiver, channeling musical energy from an invisible source.

The difficulty in achieving such freedom of expression and action is that conscious thought and effort are first required when learning artificial skills, whether to hit a tennis ball with a racquet, play the guitar, tango, or give a speech. Before a person can achieve his or her poten-tial, basic structures and fundamentals must first be learned through trial and error and subsequently practiced until they become instinctive. Unfortunately, so much emphasis is placed on rigidity, structure, and form that many people get frustrated in trying to learn a skill. They end up concentrating too hard on the mechanics. It's like trying to become an artist by doing paint-by-numbers.

I mentioned in the last chapter how an overemphasis on structure caused me to abandon playing the piano. Many years later as an adult, I found out that the musical styles on piano that I enjoyed were not written out, but largely learned by ear. Although many contemporary recording artists are grounded in classical training, for every one of those, there is probably an equal number who had no formal training. There have been musicians, such as blues pianist Otis Spann and jazz guitarist George Benson, who never learned to read a note of music, yet became virtuosos on their instruments. They still had to learn some rudimentary structures—keys, chords, and the like. But for them, that was obviously not the heavy emphasis. Those maestros learned the most by observing and listening to others. Imitation is the greatest form of flattery, and that's how they developed their unique styles. They would pick up snippets and gems from others, then use those pieces to build their own ideas.

Musicians talk about what they call "muscle memory," in which the center of intelligence seems to reside within the muscles of the hands and fingers themselves. I can appreciate this concept now that I've learned to play the piano by ear. There is absolutely no need to force your mind to remember every note. Like traveling a familiar route, winding your way through a maze of streets and landmarks without getting lost, you know the unique structure and pattern of the song and where you're headed next. It just flows from there.

Probably the most important aspect of learning to play the piano in a less-structured format is learning how to relax while playing. I just had to give up worrying about mistakes, or learning parts *exactly* as I heard them. Any time I'm tired or try hard to get a part just right, I get tripped up. Huxley coined the phrase "dynamic relaxation" as the antithesis of forced effort, and to me, his phrase is another apt translation for wu wei. "Whatever the art you may wish to learn . . . combine relaxation with activity," he wrote. "Learn to do what you have to do without strain . . . never under tension. . . . Dynamic relaxation is that state of the body and mind which is associated with normal and natural functioning."[10]

Dynamic relaxation is easy to detect in others. Even if you can't walk and chew gum at the same time, are all thumbs, or have two left feet, you are most likely immediately awestruck by the graceful movements of gifted performers. In addition to exquisite balance and coordination, the movements usually require a great deal of physical strength and stamina, but they don't appear that way to the observer—the movements look so easy. According to neurophysiologist Jonathan Cole, Russian neuropsychologist A. R. Luria "often used the term 'kinetic melody' to describe the movements of walking, dancing and running" and described how each of these acts "may be seen as melodic in its smooth and apparently effortless sliding from one phase to the next."[11] Such smooth and effortless movement is commonly called *fluid movement,* because there's nothing jerky or stilted about it—it has the quality of flowing water. According to Taoism, the closest thing in nature to pure effectiveness is, in fact, water. Huston Smith explains:

They [Taoists] were struck by the way it [water] would support objects and carry them effortlessly on its tide. The Chinese characters for swimmer, deciphered, mean literally "one who knows the nature of water." . . . In a stream [water] follows the stones' sharp edges, only to turn them into pebbles, rounded to conform to its streamlined flow. It works its way past frontiers and under dividing walls. . . . Infinitely supple, yet incomparably strong—these virtues of water are precisely those of *wu wei* as well. The person who embodies this condition . . . *acts without strain.*[12] [Emphasis added.]

The art of seeing is not an artificial skill, like that of dancing or learning to drive a car, which must be acquired through lessons and rigid training. Good vision is essential, however, for learning and excelling at many skills, activities, and crafts that are sight dependent. According to Merrill Bowan, "The purpose of vision is to guide and direct learning, and movement is its medium."[13] For us to see normally and naturally requires fluid movement. Just as strain negatively affects or hinders an artist or athlete, as explained in chapter 3, strain disrupts the fluidity and graceful motions of seeing.

GOOD VIBRATIONS

My horizon expanded one day at university. For a prairie boy who was used to seeing an endless, arching canopy of blue sky envelop the plains in all directions, my view of reality and consciousness was not so expansive. East met West for me that day in the form of a counterculture event. I was attracted out of curiosity, much like a freak show draws a crowd at the circus. A small group of young Caucasian men clad in saffron robes, each with heads shaven except for a small tuft of hair, were chanting some strange things outside in the open area where rock bands were normally set up for entertainment from time to time. "Hare Krishna, Hare Krishna, Hare Krishna," they chanted, accompanied by simple percussion instruments.

The chanting eventually stopped after a few minutes, and the group spokesperson grabbed the microphone to explain what they were doing and what they represented. If I had closed my eyes, I wouldn't have believed it was one of these strange-looking chanters; he actually sounded like a regular Western guy. A very articulate man, he had some interesting thoughts about the negativity of Western consumerism and materialism. My friends and I quickly tuned out, however, and made jibes among ourselves about these guys probably being a bunch of former hippie burnouts who were now getting high on this weird Eastern mysticism. There we were, applying ourselves in school to embark eventually on engineering careers in society. Were these guys going to live like monks for the rest of their lives? How practical was that? Maybe they had the last laugh.

This was the decade after the turbulent sixties. The hippies, with their "Make love, not war" motto—rejecting the aggressive ways of materialism, environmental destruction, and senseless warfare—had ironically been on a self-destructive path with their mind-altering drugs and hedonistic lifestyles. A turning point occurred when Beatle George Harrison produced the single "Hare Krishna Mantra." Once the song hit the pop charts, Krishna all of a sudden went from obscure to well-known. Because other seeds of Eastern consciousness had also been germinating in North America, the result was an overwhelming shift in awareness in modern society.

The "Age of Aquarius" had dawned, and the cultural phenomena were later dubbed "New Age." Many prominent Western writers, poets, scientists, and politicians in the nineteenth and early twentieth centuries had dabbled in the study of Eastern philosophies and religions, so the New Age concepts in the sixties were hardly new. The difference was the alternative viewpoints that exploded on the scene. But hippie idealism gave way to pragmatism; progress and the rat race were here to stay, and very few were willing to sacrifice their lives to become ascetics. Perhaps there was a way to have the best of both worlds—one foot in the East and one foot in the West. Big business became fashionable again with the ensuing "yuppie" years, and the New Age was everywhere, from the legitimate and useful to the crass and flaky.

Decades before the tremors of the New Age had begun to reverberate, Selye's work had caused another type of quake in the medical sciences. His research findings on the stress syndrome spawned huge interest in the study of stress as it related to health and disease. Negative emotions were found to be the biggest stressors; and as discussed in the previous chapter, that commodity is still all too commonplace in our high-tech times. Whether the pace exerts intense pressure, or the career situation is just plain frustrating, the emotional strain wreaks havoc. Conventional wisdom and relaxation methods were the foundation for a host of New Age consciousness techniques to help people better cope with distress and thereby limit the strain to their health. Selye's *The Stress of Life,* originally published in 1956, was updated in 1976 partly in response to the massive cultural shift and interest in Eastern antidotes to the rat race.

Two of the most important conventional relaxation methods were finding happiness in work and having diversionary activities aside from work. Finding enjoyable life work has long been a goal for young people. George Bernard Shaw had said, "Labor is doing what we must; leisure is doing what we like." Or, as Robert Frost put it:

> My object in living is to unite
> My avocation and my vocation
> As my two eyes make one in sight.[14]

With the mounting data on the ill effects of stress and strain, finding career contentment eventually became a matter of health. An ounce of prevention is the idea behind aptitude tests, which are designed to help match a person's natural talents with certain careers to avoid the pitfall of lifelong frustration.

If people weren't lucky enough to find work that was paid play or the perfect fit, the importance of diversionary activities, interests, and hobbies were emphasized. "A change is as good as a rest" has been medically verified. But it can't just be idle time off, for, as Selye observed, "Nothing to do is not to rest; a vacant mind and a slothful body suffer the distress of deprivation."[15] The new Eastern methods then came along, offering a veritable potpourri of relaxing diversions from the rigors of life.

Science recognized the efficacy of the many new offerings but was largely reluctant to accept the spiritual, mystical, or higher-consciousness aspects. Some, like Selye, weren't concerned about such associations, but with the caveat that matter was divorced from mind: "The biologic mechanism of all these practices remains to be clarified," Selye noted.[16] For others, much of the New Age methodology was watered down—capturing the nuts and bolts of what could be conceived as real—to make it more acceptable and palatable to a society steeped in techno-logical advances. The proponents and practitioners certainly didn't want to be viewed as being part of cults or reverting back to superstition. So instead of practicing meditation, people practiced the Relaxation Response, progressive relaxation, or a form of self-hypnosis. Spirit or soul was the subliminal mind or the subconscious. Yoga involved muscle flexibility and deep-breathing exercises. Martial arts were just another form of physical fitness.

The ancient practices of yoga and meditation actually weave their way through several Eastern cultures and countries. There are offshoots and differences, but there also are many common threads. Certain sects of Taoism have practiced many of these ancient traditions, with the aim of maximizing *ch'i,* the mysterious vital energy or life force. The tech-niques all sought wu wei to minimize strain and friction with the self, others, or nature. They included yogic breathing, meditation, and grace-ful motion, such as the art of tai ch'i.

The ancient tradition that continues to fascinate Westerners is medi-tation, now a household word. It may now be eclectic mainstream, a type of "mind exercise" intended to provide short-term benefits like a burst of energy for a hectic workday as well as the long-term benefit of improved health. Even if you find the spiritual, religious, and mystical roots hard to swallow, I think it's important not to ignore the thou-sands of years of history and the true aim of meditators, from Taoists, to Zen Buddhists, to Hare Krishna followers. The chants and the mantras are sounds generated by the individual, repeated in a rhythmic fashion. Contrary to what some people think, it's not about sitting totally still with a blank mind. It's movement at the most ephemeral and subtle level, an intensely centered internal focus, connecting directly to a supreme vibra-tion. Those who have attained a state of altered consciousness claim to have temporarily transcended our material trappings, hence the name Transcendental Meditation for one popular technique. The transcenden-tal condition is a brief respite to counteract the anxieties and negative emotions built up by conscious striving. Regardless of the means, it's all about good vibrations.

THE HEALTH BEAT

"Pa rum-pum-pum-pum." It seems the Little Drummer Boy knew a good thing when he tapped on his drum. If "laughter is the best medicine," then the joy of music I mentioned in chapter 3 appears to elicit a similar healthy outcome.

Probably the most fundamental form of musical rhythm is drumming. Having endured centuries of "civilization" imposed upon them by North American settlers, the aboriginal people in my home province have managed to save one of their most sacred traditions, the pow-wow. (Unfortunately, their eyesight doesn't seem to have been spared, because just as high a percentage of them sport spectacles as European Canadians.) During pow-wows, the indigenous people gather in a circle to partake in a very special and rhythmic event. Dressed in beautiful ceremonial attire, members of the community dance in intricate moves synchronized with the continual beat and chanting of the drummers. The rich, dynamic heritage and potent sense of higher meaning are palpable to outside observers.

Modern society, which once ridiculed the pow-wow as wild and crazy, is ironically now using drumming circles as a form of health therapy. Dr. Barry Bittman, a Pittsburgh neurologist, has offered drumming "as a therapeutic intervention to . . . patients suffering from some of the most challenging illnesses imaginable . . . cancer, heart disease, chronic lung disease and diabetes."[17] The very act of pounding on drums in unison with others apparently has a harmonizing and calming effect on our many internal body rhythms; sound, music, and vibration evoke strong responses from the systems and cells of the human body.[18] There are definite and measurable physiological changes that lower stress levels and boost the immune system. Bittman elaborates eloquently:

Deep within the essence of who we are there's a sound, a vibration, an emanation that expresses life from every cell. It resonates in harmony with all living creatures—an inner voice ready to emerge as a vital heartbeat that inscribes a personal signature.

The rhythm of life is a symphony—the expression of our soul

revealed by the conductor within. Our unique voice resounds through the way we choose to live. When we connect with each other and extend ourselves to one another, we share our gift.

When our hands connect with a drum that vibrates with our energy, vitality, emotion, exhilaration, hope sensitivity, giving, sharing and unity, we become whole again. . . . Group drumming opens doors, enhances self-esteem, ensures a healthy workout, stimulates our minds, boosts our creative potential, makes us laugh and connects us on many levels. It also builds bridges, heightens awareness and strengthens bonds. . . . Group drumming tunes our biology, orchestrates our immunity, and enables healing to begin.[19]

There are now many trained drumming facilitators who conduct group workshops and sessions—not just for people with serious health problems, but also for members of the general public who are looking for an alternative diversion to the daily grind, hoping to tap into something beyond the superficial and mundane. Participants describe these sessions as being equally exhilarating and deeply relaxing. Rhythm is at the very core of our existence, and the effect of drumming seems to be very primal, connecting directly to people's souls. The beat goes on, and healthy vision is certainly no exception.

EYESIGHT R&R

Long before all the interest in stress and how to relax for optimum health and peak performance, Bates was way ahead of the game. Once he discovered that strain caused blurred vision, he concluded such an unnatural state could be reversed, and possibly even totally eliminated. The way to go about effecting such an improvement had to be rest and relaxation (R&R), and this is where we come to the third primary fact of his teachings:

> Perfect sight can be obtained only by relaxation. Nothing else matters.[20]

Fair enough. So, why isn't it just a matter of getting a few nights of good sleep to reverse eyestrain? To this Bates had responded, "The eyes are rarely, if ever, completely relaxed in sleep, and if they are under a strain when the subject is awake, that strain will certainly be continued during sleep, to a greater or less degree, just as a strain of other parts of the body is continued."[21] What about avoiding close work or other activities that supposedly strain the eyes during the day? Bates's reply to this notion: "The idea that it rests the eyes not to use them is also erroneous."[22] On the surface, these are seemingly strange concepts about rest and relaxation; sleep doesn't rest the eyesight, nor does avoidance of eye use for certain close activities during the day.

Actually Bates's notions aren't so strange. Eye movements and focusing consist of several different muscles acting in complex and mysterious harmony. Medical science knows that chronically contracted (tense) muscles in other parts of the body work continuously, and the constant tension never leaves even when sleeping.[23] Contracted eye muscles are no different. As well, manifestations of work-related stressors can persist even on days off. "Simple rest is no cure-all," Hans Selye insisted. "Activity and rest must be judiciously balanced."[24] The type of relaxation Bates advocated was precisely the pure effectiveness and fluid movement previously discussed. Quiet the conscious strain and mental effort in conjunction with proper movement to achieve more efficient functioning.

F. M. Alexander, a Shakespearean performer in the late 1800s, found out that rest by avoidance didn't help his vocal problems. He began to suffer difficulties that threatened to end his chosen profession; he developed an acute case of *aphonia*—a loss of voice to all but a whisper. The advice from medical doctors was to rest his voice and speak as little as possible between performances. Alexander followed the doctors' orders to the letter, but to no avail. As soon as he returned to the stage and began projecting his voice, the symptoms would recur about an hour later. After several rest periods between performances, Alexander began to wonder if his throat problems resulted from an improper use of his voice. Perhaps he was straining his throat, because other performers didn't suffer the problem. But what was he doing wrong?

That question, and the ultimate answer, led to what is now the world-renowned Alexander Technique. Through trial and error and hours of personal observation in a mirror, Alexander discovered he tensed up in several faulty postural positions that reduced the efficiency of his voice. Even though the positions felt normal to him, according to Alexander Technique teacher Glynn MacDonald, "he began to realize that the mirror was informing him of movements he had not been aware of making, and that he could not trust his feelings." His body feedback hadn't been telling him that he was straining, but now he could clearly see it. The strain had become habitual and suppressed from his awareness, but it ultimately manifested itself as throat symptoms. Once he understood what he was doing wrong, he had to break the old habits and consciously learn the proper habits. "The inflammation of the vocal cords disappeared and his voice became reliable and effective," MacDonald says. "His general health also improved."[25]

A change may be as good as a rest, but as both F. M. Alexander and Bates discovered in their own ways, it can't be just any kind of change. People have to understand, said Bates, that the change must be proper: "This relaxation cannot, however, be obtained by any sort of effort . . . for so long as they think, consciously or unconsciously, that relief from strain may be obtained by another strain their cure [improvement] will be delayed."[26] The relaxation Bates was encouraging was essentially much like Alexander's—poised and fluid movement. But the difficulty with vision is that people have trouble studying their own incorrect movements. It generally requires the experienced observation of someone who understands and teaches Bates's techniques.

The concept of "relearning to see" is the premise of Tom Quackenbush's entire NVI program. He teaches movement as the first principle and says that one must practice correct vision habits to undo years of strain that caused and maintained the blurred vision.[27] In essence, people with blurry vision have become addicted to seeing with strain and effort; they've forgotten how to see naturally. Aldous Huxley stated that good vision "may subsequently be consciously reacquired by anyone who has learned the suitable techniques. When it has been reacquired, the strain associated with impaired functioning disappears and the organs involved [the eyes] do their work in a condition of dynamic relaxation."[28] You just need to be taught how to snap out of your visual amnesia and begin to wean yourself from your addictive ways. Softness, fluid movements, and good vibrations—that's our next chapter.

5
RETURN

Returning is the motion of the Tao.
Yielding is the way of the Tao.

Now things grow profusely,
Each again returns to its root.
To return to the root is to attain quietude.

Seeing the small is called clarity;
keeping flexible is called strength.
Using the shining radiance,
you return again to the light.

LAO TZU[1]

Speaking of returns, have you ever watched professional tennis players compete? The player awaiting the opponent's serve is in continual motion, briskly dancing about on the balls of his or her feet, rocking from side to side, all the while twirling the racket. In the heat of competition, the athletes are geared up with nervous energy, so it makes sense that they want to stay agile to keep their muscles loose. But you'd think all this movement would be distracting once the opponent tosses the ball up before striking it. Why doesn't the player awaiting the serve just stand still at that point and watch carefully? It may seem paradoxical, but it's precisely the seemingly fidgety movements that intensify their focus.

Professional tennis players are able to serve the ball at speeds in excess of 130 miles per hour. A ball being served at that rate takes only about half a second to reach the receiving player. Keen eyesight is absolutely crucial under these circumstances. Howard Brody, longtime tennis researcher and retired physics professor, says tennis players who are skilled at returning serves "have incredibly good eyesight."[2] Without knowing it, tennis players are practicing Bates's techniques for relaxed eye movement. In tennis instruction, the body motion while awaiting the serve is called the *rock,* constantly transferring weight from one leg to the other and back again. While rocking, players are also taught to alternate looking down to the ground, then back up to the opponent. In NVI terms, these two things are called the *sway* and the *shift.* The pros also unknowingly practice a type of mental shift, as tennis star Andy Roddick confirms: "[It's] important . . . to stay quick mentally. If you get discouraged . . . then the serves start flying past you. . . . You have to be able to focus on every one, so you can't get down about one that gets away from you."[3] He avoids mental locking—replaying in his mind's eye the one he was just unable to return.

This chapter outlines Bates's key fundamentals and techniques that have helped many people return to naturally clear vision. If you have blurred vision, you must stay mobile and "dodge the stare" to have any hope of reversing the tension built up in your eye muscles from years of strain.

FUNDAMENTALS OF CLEAR SIGHT

There is a plethora of books, audiotapes, videos, and infomercials in the marketplace targeted at those wishing to achieve greater financial success and career achievement in our highly materialistic society. What do most of these sources have in common? The purveyors of the success business have usually studied what has worked for famous role models, and then captured a few practices or consistent habits of those who've made it.

I suppose Bates was in the success business long before it became fashionable. In a similar vein, he identified key things that people with excellent sight do unconsciously and continually. Before embarking on any of Bates's relaxed-vision techniques, it is imperative to fully understand and consciously be aware of these fundamentals. Note that, for all intents and purposes, they essentially *all happen concurrently;* they are separated only for the purpose of explaining them. Shifting and blinking are two fundamentals that are not difficult to understand, but they must be done properly. You may find the other two—consciousness of apparent movement (the swing) and concentric focus—to be tricky and subtle concepts to comprehend at first, but I emphasize, *do not underestimate their importance in the least.*

> The fundamentals of clear sight must be practiced at all times. . . . The normal eye does these things unconsciously and the imperfect eye must at first practice them consciously until it becomes an unconscious habit.[4]

Quackenbush is of the view that these statements "are possibly the . . . most important . . . ever written about improving eyesight naturally."[5] I couldn't agree more. That's why I consider these concepts so vital to success with NVI. Let's discuss each:

Shifting

Someone with shifty eyes is not to be trusted. In Western culture, it's considered impolite and even suspicious not to look a person in the eyes during conversation. If someone keeps looking away, that individual is thought to have something to hide. It's too bad "shifty eyes" has such a negative connotation, because that's exactly what you need for good vision. The shifts need not be so large, however; you can still be polite and maintain eye contact while continually and inconspicuously shifting. Here's what Bates had to say about the importance of shifting:

It is impossible for the eye to fix a point longer than a fraction of a second. If it tries to do so, it begins to strain and the vision is lowered. This can readily be demonstrated by trying to hold one part of a letter for an appreciable length of time. No matter how good the sight, it will begin to blur, or even disappear, very quickly, and sometimes the effort to hold it will produce pain. In the case of a few exceptional people a point may appear to be held for a considerable length of time; the subjects themselves may think that they are holding it; but this is only because the eye shifts unconsciously, the movements being so rapid that objects seem to be seen all alike simultaneously. The shifting of the eye with normal vision is usually not conspicuous, but by direct examination . . . is seen to move in various directions, from side to side, up and down in an orbit which is usually variable.[6]

Vision science confirms that regarding a point indeed lasts only a fraction of a second, normally about 200 to 300 milliseconds, before the eyes move on to another point. That means the eyes shift focus about three to five times a second. But note, we once again encounter a problem with our static language in a dynamic world. Phraseology such as *holding* or *fixating* your gaze, even though the act is incredibly short in duration, suggests the eye temporarily goes into a freeze-frame mode. Yet it doesn't. During the time the attention is momentarily on a point between shifts, the eye remains in motion. Recall from chapter 3, eye tremors—the microvibrations that help keep the image clearly centered—cycle thirty to seventy times a second. Presumably Bates had a hunch that something as fast as tremors did exist, because he stated, "The eye is capable of shifting with a rapidity which the ophthalmoscope [an instrument used to give a closeup view of the eye and retina] cannot measure."[7] So instead of *fixating* in between shifts, I prefer to simply say *focusing*, even though it's technically not the correct term.

The shifts Bates was perhaps observing were the various other types of eye movements categorized by modern vision science, movements such as *saccades* (also called *jumps*), *pursuit tracking*, or *smooth tracking*. Whether the tracking motions or jumps are detectable to an observer with or without the aid of an instrument, the eye is continually changing and adapting its focus by means of shifting. In their book *Total Vision*, Richard Kavner and Loraine Dusky confirm the importance of continual shifting:

> A perfect eye continually wiggles. . . . [It] is in constant motion, oscillating from side to side. This slight but constant movement is normally imperceptible. In one experiment, a special contact lens was rigged up to keep the image stabilized as if the eye did not move. Within a minute, the subject experienced a loss of vision. . . . The eye needs to be always on the go, looking here, looking there, picking out what it wants, what it can't help noticing, and shuffling all this information around. . . . Become "fixed" on something to the exclusion of new data, and you lose your perspective.[8]

Taoists understand this concept as a general principle. Referring to any attempt at control in nature, Lao Tzu had said, "If you try to hold it, you will lose it."[9] Consequently, proper shifting means a healthy refractive rhythm. But the dynamics of vision aren't just in these outward movements. Neurobiological researchers have recently confirmed that the inward receiving aspect of our vision is also in flux. The visual cortex in the brain doesn't have static "receptive domains" as was once thought, but "dynamic fields of integration and association."[10] Even down to the microscopic level, visual cells are dynamic. Any strain or effort that disrupts the shifting has a serious consequence on the eye's refractive dynamics.

For those of you with blurred vision, don't expect to regain proper shifting of the eyes in short order. Bates found that people who began to improve their eyesight by means of relaxation invariably strained if they attempted to consciously shift too rapidly. That's why he and subsequent instructors developed many methods and techniques to help people gradually reacquire the natural rapid shifting. It's somewhat like learning cursive writing in school, when you first had to learn how to write slowly in bigger and more pronounced motions. Several of the relaxed eye-movement methods are discussed later in the chapter. For now, the benefit of this fundamental cannot be overstated. "It is only when the eye is able to shift . . . rapidly," Bates wrote, "that eye and mind are at rest, and the efficiency of both at their maximum. . . . Perfect sight is impossible without continual shifting."[11] The shorter and more rapid the shifts, the better.

Apparent Movement (The Swing)

A local radio talk-show host speaking about politics one day said, "Perception is reality." He was responding to a caller bemoaning the way the electorate seems to vote out of fear rather than carefully weighing a logically and positively presented platform. Sales and Marketing 101—sell the sizzle, not the steak. People make decisions based on emotions, not logic. So whether it's voting for a candidate to prevent pain or buying a product for pleasure, what you perceive will happen is your reality at that moment.

"Perception is reality" is also an apt description for optical illusions. You may think you're seeing lines bending, when in fact they're actually parallel; or you'll see shapes of different sizes when they're really identical. We're tricked by a perceived reality. Optical illusions usually occur when there is a clash of two different perspectives, either side by side or overlapping. Our eyes and mind tend to merge the data, giving us mixed signals.

Seeing apparent movement, or a swing, is an optical illusion that people with good vision experience, usually without knowing it. When you shift your focus and attention from one point to another, you immediately shift your perspective. To see what I mean, here's a simple demonstration you can try. Close your left eye and place your index finger directly in the line of your right eye's central vision about a foot away. While glancing at your finger with your right eye, use your peripheral vision to note a background object a few feet away that's almost in line with your finger. Now open your left eye to look directly at the background object while simultaneously closing your right eye. The finger should now be in the peripheral field of your left eye.

Notice what happened to your finger? If you did this properly, you should have had the illusion that it "jumped" or "moved" to the right even though it was stationary. Try it again in an alternating fashion with each eye, right, left, right, left, in quick succession. Hopefully you'll be able to do this successfully to get the sensation of the finger swinging back and forth. If not, don't worry about it for now; it means you're straining, and there's no point in continuing the strain.

What really happened in this little demonstration? Your right eye's central vision first saw your finger head on, while your left eye's peripheral vision next saw it off to the right, two completely different angles, or perspectives, in space. As you alternate, or shift, your perspective from left eye to right eye and back again, the stationary finger magically appears to swing back and forth. Obviously this demonstration is no way to use your eyes for coordinated vision. Relaxed vision also requires head and neck movement in concert with eye movement. So, let's consider a more realistic and everyday change in perspective.

Basic math and geometry verify the change in perspective when one is reading a document. Three overly simplifying assumptions are made here: (1) the document is a foot away from you; (2) a line of text is seven inches from left margin to right margin; (3) the midpoint between your eyes is in line with the left quadrant of the page. (Note I'm not suggesting this is the proper alignment for reading. The assumptions are made merely to demonstrate.) Your first shift to begin reading is a split-second focus on the first letter at the left margin. That letter is actually a smidgen farther away (0.1 inch) than the one-foot distance of the page head-on. At that same instant, the last letter at the right margin is 13.1 inches away at an angle of 32 degrees in your right peripheral field of vision. An inch difference may not seem like much, but for focusing it's significant. Next, you smoothly shift to the right across the text. By the time you get to the right margin, the left margin is still 12.1 inches away, but it's now in your left peripheral field at an angle of 32 degrees. At the end of the line, you shift rapidly back to the left margin of the next lower line to repeat the smooth shifting process again. Perspective and focus keep changing constantly at all points between the two margins.

Compare that scenario to reading an eye chart from a distance. Aside from the performance anxiety of being tested, checking vision in this manner encourages the strain of staring. You are standing or sitting still with virtually no head or neck movement. Instead of smooth tracking, the eyes are forced to pause too long at each letter. Stopping the macromovements of shifting to hold your gaze impairs the micromovements of shifting. If a letter is a bit blurry, then the person strains to try and bring it in clearly. But the effort backfires. The key to seeing the individual letters without staring is continual small shifts, which in turn elicit the illusion of small apparent swings.

> When the eye with normal vision regards a letter either at the near-point or at a distance, the letter may appear to pulsate, or to move in various directions, from side to side, up and down, or obliquely. When it looks from one letter to another on the Snellen test card [eye chart], or from one side of a letter to another, not only the letter, but the whole line of letters and the whole card, may appear to move from side to side. This apparent movement is due to the shifting of the eye, and is always in a direction contrary to its movement. If one looks at the top of a letter, the letter is below the line of vision, and, therefore, appears to move downward. If one looks at the bottom, the letter is above the line of vision and appears to move upward. If one looks to the left of the letter, it is to the right of the line of vision and appears to move to the right. If one looks to the right, it is to the left of the line of vision and appears to move to the left.
>
> Persons with normal vision are rarely conscious of this illusion, and may have difficulty in demonstrating it; but in every case that has come under my observation they have always become able, in a longer or shorter time, to do so. When the sight is imperfect the letters may remain stationary, or even move in the same direction as the eye.[12]

This contrary apparent movement is also called *oppositional movement* by contemporary NVI instructors. Whenever you shift your focus with your eyes and head, stationary objects in your peripheral field should have the appearance of moving in the opposite direction. The swing, then, is a *reaction* to the first fundamental, the shift, as Bates notes: "The eye can shift voluntarily. This is a muscular act resulting from a motor impulse. But the swing comes of its own accord when the shifting is normal."[13] It follows, then, that the more rapid and short the shift, the more subtle the illusion of the swing. A further corollary follows that the shorter and quicker the illusion of the swing, the more relaxed the vision. The ability to see the illusion of the swing of a single small-font letter when shifting from one side to the other is most likely impossible for those with blurred vision. As with relearning how to shift, you must build gradually by learning techniques to start seeing the illusion of longer and slower swings.

It wasn't until I better understood the swing and its significance that I concluded that my first flash of clear vision very early in my NVI journey occurred because of it. When I was walking home that day without wearing glasses, I reached the end of the block and proceeded to turn to the left on the sidewalk. As I rounded the corner, my eyes, head, and body motion were flowing left while the house and fence on the corner across from me swung to the right, in the opposite direction. The flash occurred once I'd completely rounded the corner—boom, just like that. The opposing apparent movement, even though I wasn't conscious of it at the time, was enough to temporarily relax my eyes for those few brief seconds.

After I'd finally made the connection between the swing and flash, the many more flashes that continued to come generally involved similar types of motion, whereby objects in my peripheral field would move in the contrary direction. I also then realized why my wife has such good vision. Considered extremely hyper because she can barely sit still, she's in continual motion all day long. (My university training taught me there's no such thing as a perpetual-motion machine. Oh, yeah? I married one!) Having an analytical and methodical bent, I'm a long way from becoming hyper. But I sure try to move much more now, even subtly when sitting, to consciously get the illusion of the swing.

Concentric Focus

When you drop a stone into a quiet pond of water, you get a familiar pattern. A series of concentric waves emerges from the center and continues outward. The wave is strongest at the center in response to the energy transfer from the stone crashing through the surface. The waves gradually slow down and dissipate the farther they get from the center. Michael Colebrook of GreenSpirit suggests, "It could be claimed that the human sensory system was designed specifically to provide awareness of emergent phenomena."[14] This could certainly be said for our sense of sight. The anatomy of the eye is such that the light receptors in back of the eye (retina) are distributed in a concentric pattern to see rays emerging from the object at the point of attention. Bates wrote:

> Minute rodlike and conical bodies . . . vary in form and are distributed very differently in its different parts. In the center of the retina . . . there are no rods, and the cones are elongated and pressed very closely together. . . . Beyond the center . . . the cones become thicker and fewer and are interspersed with rods, the number of which increases toward the margin of the retina. The precise function of these rods and cones is not clear; but it is a fact that the center . . . where all elements except the cones and their associated cells practically disappear, is the seat of the most acute vision. As we withdraw from this spot, the acuteness of the visual perceptions rapidly decreases. The eye with normal vision, therefore, sees one part of everything it looks at best, and everything else worse, in proportion as it is removed from the point of maximum vision.[15]

Modern vision science has a better understanding of the role of cones and rods. For a more detailed explanation and diagrams of their distribution pattern, refer to chapter 17 in Tom Quackenbush's *Relearning to See*. Because of this anatomical fact, Bates called the phenomenon *central fixation*. As noted in the previous section, the term *fixation* presents a problem in that it may be interpreted as regarding a point of interest too long, at which stage it becomes a stare and a strain. Contemporary

NVI instructors have substituted phrases such as *nuclear vision* and *centralization* to avoid the danger of the stare when learning this fundamental. I've chosen to coin the phrase *concentric focus* for two reasons: the concentric anatomical distribution of light receptors gives us the clearest sight in the center, gradually diminishing in clarity toward the periphery; and our focus is dynamic, much like the concentric waves in the pond.

Mental strain has the effect of impairing this concentric focus, an inverse condition Bates called *eccentric fixation*. In this case I will not alter the phrase, because a person is fixating, or staring, to get this negative effect:

> When the vision of the center of sight has been suppressed, partially or completely, the patient can no longer see the point which he is looking at best, but sees objects not regarded directly as well, or better, because the sensitiveness of the retina has now become approximately equal in every part, or is even better in the outer part than in the center. Therefore in all cases of defective vision the patient is unable to see best where he is looking. . . . Eccentric fixation, even in its lesser degrees, is so unnatural that great discomfort, or even pain, can be produced in a few seconds by trying to see every part of an area three or four inches in extent at twenty feet, or even less, or an area of an inch or less at the near-point, equally well at one time.[16]

Besides the anatomical fact of concentric focus, there is another reason why eccentric fixation is impossible and a strain. Consider a similar example as discussed with the fundamental of the swing. This time assume the text is on a computer monitor a foot away, and your line of sight is in the exact center of the screen. Imagine you are regarding a single letter at that point, again by rapidly shifting and swinging the letter. Once again, we use basic math and geometry to find that the farther the peripheral vision is from the center, the farther away the text is from the eyes. The eye is focused for one point only, the center letter. The peripheral concentric "rings" of vision are farther and farther away, so they will automatically be more and more out of focus while you still regard the center letter. Think of it like a target. The bull's eye is 12 inches from the midpoint between your eyes, but for concentric circles of diameters 4, 8, and 12 inches, the text at those points will be 12.2, 12.6, and 13.4 inches away.

What we have here is a consequence of the drab straight lines, squares, and rectangles that clutter the landscape of our literate world. We read on flat, two-dimensional (2D) paper, computer monitors, black-boards, and projection screens. On the other hand, the outside world of nature is ablaze with three-dimensional (3D) magnificence and splendor. When people strain to read, do they somehow suppress the concentric focus, subconsciously thinking a flat medium is equidistant from the eyes wherever they look? Whatever the cause, eccentric fixation means blurred vision.

Prescription lenses for myopia, when worn to read, perpetuate the problem of eccentric fixation. You may very well be seeing too much area clearly all at once. This clearness before you actually becomes flat-tened; you get artificial 2D vision at the expense of sensing depth of field. Almost as stunning as experiencing the flash of clear vision for the first time was seeing 3D again. What I soon started to notice with clear flashes of vision outside was the incredible depth perception. I thought I was seeing 3D with glasses on before, but it was an illusion. I must have been subconsciously judging depth of field by the size of familiar objects. The difference between perceived 3D and natural 3D is unmistakable. I never thought I'd look at leaves on a tree with such wonder and amaze-ment. The richness of the sharpest green you could imagine on part of a leaf being looked at in the center of vision, combined with amazing depth perception of the peripheral branches and leaves, is stunning.

As Lao Tzu said, seeing the small is indeed clarity. Just how small is the centermost clear spot of vision with concentric focus? Infinitesimal, according to Bates:

> Contrary to what is generally believed, the part seen best when the sight is normal is extremely small. The text-books say that at

twenty feet an area having a diameter of half an inch can be seen with maximum vision, but anyone who tries at this distance to see every part of even the smallest letters of the Snellen test card—the diameter of which may be less than a quarter of an inch—equally well at one time will immediately become myopic. The fact is that the nearer the point of maximum vision approaches a mathematical point, which has no area, the better the sight.[17]

There's a rather paradoxical concept. You see best where there is no area! Actually, for practical purposes let's say your field consists of 0.1 percent central vision and 99.9 percent peripheral vision. Concentric focus may be an obscure fact, but it's one that can be readily demonstrated. The *Encarta* encyclopedia states, "Subjectively, a person is not conscious that the visual field consists of a central zone of sharpness surrounded by an area of increasing fuzziness. The reason is that the eyes are constantly moving . . . as the attention is shifted from one object to another."[18] Those with good vision can, if consciously aware of this fundamental fact of concentric focus, observe that only a tiny spot in the center is clearest. But for those with visual blur, as with the first two fundamentals, this ability has to be regained gradually.

Blinking

In his earlier works on improving vision naturally, Bates did not devote much attention to the discussion of blinking for good vision. In subsequent years, however, he emphasized the significance of proper blinking in numerous issues of his journal, *Better Eyesight*. For this reason, I have included blinking as the fourth key fundamental.

As noted in chapter 3, blinking is a rapid and involuntary reflex of the eyelids opening and closing an average of fifteen to thirty times a minute. One of the main purposes of blinking is to keep our eyes lubricated with a protective tear layer and to keep refreshing the layer by washing away dust or fine particles that make contact with the surface. It has been suggested that another reason for blinking is to temporarily close off light to the eyes every few seconds. But as far as Bates was concerned, the most important purpose of blinking is to avoid staring. The eyes shift every time we blink, even during sleep. So in that sense, blinking is directly related to the first fundamental.

In 1925 Bates wrote, "Blinking is very important. It is not the brief periods of rest obtained from closing the eyes which helps the sight so much as the shifting or movements of the eyes. It should be repeatedly demonstrated that the eyes are only at rest when they are shifting."[19] Two years later he added, "It can always be demonstrated that when a patient with imperfect sight looks intently at one point, keeping the eyes open constantly, or trying to do so, that a strain of the eyes and all the nerves of the body is usually felt, and the vision becomes imperfect. It is impossible to keep the eyes open continuously without blinking. Each time the eyes blink, a certain amount of rest is obtained and the vision is benefitted."[20]

Although blinking is involuntary, the blink rate is impaired by strain. But what makes blinking more than just shifting, though, is the protective cleansing action, because the eyes dry out with insufficient blinking, leading to redness, irritation, and possible lowering of the vision. With the widespread use of computers nowadays, people are warned of the dangers of eyestrain, particularly "dry eye syndrome." The sensations may include burning, stinging, or grittiness. The condition is actually fairly common, with estimates of up to 28 percent incidence among the adult population. Studies have verified that eyestrain associated with computer work and intense near work results in much less frequent blinking. Staring and concentration can reduce the blink rate by half to two thirds. That means some people are blinking only four to seven times a minute when concentrating.[21]

If blinking frequently is good for your vision, is a higher blink rate even better? From an NVI perspective, no. During moments of nervousness and high pressure, the blink frequency increases dramatically. In the 1996 United States presidential debates, according to David Givens of the Center for Nonverbal Studies, "candidate Bob Dole averaged 147 blinks—seven times above normal. President Bill Clinton averaged 99 blinks a minute, reaching 117 when asked about increases in teen drug use, a sensitive issue of the day."[22] These were only temporary changes under adverse conditions. Can you imagine the eyestrain if this type of rapid blinking went on continuously?* Bates's teachings suggest that blinking too fast is as bad as not blinking enough. When people "acquire the habit of blinking too fast, they are very apt to stare while they blink," he observed. The eyelids must not open or close shut too quickly with a nervous twitch that may cause more strain; "blink one blink at a time," he recommended, "instead of blinking rapidly."[23]

To dodge the stare and keep your eyes properly moistened and protected, it's imperative to remember to blink frequently throughout the day, particularly when doing intense work involving much mental effort. Even in more favorable conditions, it's also important. In the brighter natural light of the sun outdoors, we may be tempted to not blink enough because the vision is better than under dimmer artificial lighting. We may have the tendency to strain to bring things into focus even better, or to hold onto flashes of clear vision without blinks.

Blinking every couple of seconds during regular eye-shifting needs to be consciously cultivated to restore a healthy and natural blink reflex. It is also important that no strain be associated with the blinking action itself. The opening and closing must be soft. "When blinking [people] may fail to obtain relaxation," Bates said, "because they too often blink with an effort. . . . Shifting of the eyes up and down improves the vision, when blinking is done easily, without effort."[24]

To reiterate, these four fundamentals are separated solely for the purpose of discussion and explanation. Refractive rhythm is a constant dynamic interplay. Each time you shift your attention from one point to the next, the swing causes apparent movement of the first point in the counter direction. While on each point for a split second, the concentric focus

---

*There is a rare eye-spasm disorder, called blepharospasm, that causes an excessive blink rate due to involuntary contractions of the muscles around the eyes. The cause of this neurological condition is not known, but it is interesting to note that the spasms are often brought on by bright lights, extended time reading, or extreme stress. The increased blink rate and spasms leave many sufferers functionally blind.

brings in the small point of attention most clearly relative to everything else in the peripheral view. Blinking need not be done on every shift, for that would be unnaturally rapid. The blinks should be done softly every couple of seconds or so.

All this advice may sound straightforward, but it's not easy to do if you have blurred vision. If it were that simple, there would be no need to learn anything else but the fundamentals. The soft overcomes the hard, but the hard is darn stubborn. That's why relaxation techniques were developed to help people reacquire the fundamentals of naturally clear sight. The idea is to return to the fundamentals consciously and gradually until they can again become unconscious and effortless.

BATES'S INSIGHT

Is your belly button an innie or an outie? I don't have to ask you such a personal question about your eyes, because they see in two ways. Our eyes actively see both our outside world, which we call *reality*, and our rich inner landscape of dreams and imagination. We discount this inner world as not being real. For example, you'll awaken from a nightmare and exclaim, "Thank God it was *only* a dream!" The imagined danger no longer threatens you because it's not outer reality, but your physiological reaction was the same. You may have screamed and sat bolt upright. You were likely sweating, while your heart beat rapidly and your breathing was shallow. Not only did you see this scary inner world but you also experienced it fully; so in that sense, it was very real.

On occasion, some get stuck between the inner and outer worlds; we call this *sleepwalking*. When he was preschool age, our oldest boy used to get up and walk about the hallway crying, obviously in terror. It was spooky for us as parents the first time it happened. My wife and I consoled him to try and settle him down. It became quickly apparent that he wasn't awake, but only seemed awake. His eyes were open but had a distant, glazed look, and he wasn't responding to our voices and touch assuring him everything was okay. He would continue to cry and babble, as if speaking in tongues. About the only discernible word he would shout out now and again would be "No!" Whatever he was dreaming, it was absolutely terrifying, as he was fully immersed in the netherworld. After about five to ten minutes, he calmed down and came out of the trancelike state, somewhat lucid yet puzzled why he was out of bed. He went through a stage where he had perhaps two or three sleepwalking night terrors a month, but they eventually stopped, never to recur.

When people are awake, the inner world doesn't completely shut off. It's considered sane behavior to daydream and imagine things while unconsciously carrying on some activity. If I'm really off somewhere in inner space, someone may joke, "Hello—earth to Doug!" Unfortunately, many mentally ill people can't snap out if it. They're tormented by hallucinations while awake, unable to distinguish between inner and outer reality. They are dazed and confused, doomed to a state very much like permanent sleepwalking.

Young children have incredibly active and vivid imaginations, yet we don't classify them as mad. We encourage their play-acting, free-form, and imaginary endeavors, considering their antics to be loveable and cute at this stage in their lives. The trouble is, as soon as the children get to school age, the classroom has a way of quickly shutting down and diminishing their creative energy. In fact, the once loveable and cutesy characteristics are mainly discouraged and considered immature. The children must behave and conform. There are "important" adult things to learn. Psychology author F. David Peat describes how this atmosphere smothers creativity:

> The thrill, the imagination, the play of childhood passes—although for some it never really goes. But what has happened, why does the world become so dull for some of us? Punishment and cruelty are obvious answers. And the low value that adults put on play and the high value they put on learning, knowledge, technique, seriousness and making a living.
>
> But praise and reward can be just as serious a block as punishment. . . . Seeking reward can be a significant block—knowing that something you or your friends are doing is valuable and then trying

to repeat it. Children lose the fun of painting and begin to look at what their fellows are doing—this can be an important phase in learning, or it can be the first step to becoming overcompliant to external values and rules.

As adults we have internalized authority; we have roles, models, values that are not are own, goals that are placed upon us. All this can destroy creativity . . . and cripple the mind.[25]

Albert Einstein apparently didn't learn to speak until he was about three years old, and his speech continued to be labored until about age seven. There are accounts that suggest he also did poorly in grammar school, lagging behind for his age. Because of these learning difficulties, some have speculated that Einstein may have been dyslexic, but others debate this speculation, saying the evidence isn't clear. Perhaps because of his intelligence, he may have had a tendency to tune out and become wrapped up in his own inner world, aloof and indifferent—the proverbial absentminded genius.

Regardless of how you categorize his early years, Einstein's imagination didn't dwindle. It's most likely what inspired and motivated him to see things differently. Visual imagery was an integral part of his thinking. In fact, to him visual imagery *was* thinking. As an adult he wrote that his concepts came to him in images: "Words or language, as they are written or spoken, do not seem to play any role in my mechanism of thought. . . . For me it is not dubious that our thinking goes on for the most part without use of words."[26] He is also famous for saying, "Imagination is more important than knowledge." (There is more discussion on this theme of "knowledge" in chapter 8.)

Einstein's comments would have come as no surprise to Bates. The importance of cultivating and maintaining a good imagination—the *mind's eye*—and memory, its close ally, was a significant aspect of Bates's teachings:

We see very largely with the mind, and only partly with the eyes. The phenomena of vision depend upon the mind's interpretation of

the impression upon the retina. What we see is not that impression, but our own interpretation of it. Our impressions of size, color, form and location can be demonstrated to depend upon the interpretation by the mind of the retinal picture. . . . No two persons with normal sight will get the same visual impressions from the same object; for their interpretations of the retinal picture will differ as much as their individualities differ, and when the sight is imperfect the interpretation is far more variable. It reflects, in fact, the loss of mental control which is responsible for the error of refraction. When the eye is out of focus, in short, the mind is also out of focus. . . . Imagination, memory and sight are, in fact, coincident. When one is perfect, all are perfect, and when one is imperfect, all are imperfect.[27]

Visualization has been a staple technique in sports psychology for some time now. The pros have mind-gurus as well as physical coaches to aid them in reaching their peak potential. The athletes visualize a positive outcome, and many actually play the shots and the game in their imagination—not just with the eyes, but with the other senses as well. Studies have been conducted showing that such mind practice combined with physical practice is as beneficial as strictly repetitive physical practice. The athletes and their coaches know full well that imagination, memory, and sight go together. They caught onto Bates's insight, demonstrating once again that Bates was well ahead of his time. His insight is crucial to fully appreciate the eye-relaxation techniques, since they all incorporate imagination and memory to a certain extent.

RELAXATION TECHNIQUES

When the idea of improving sight without lenses was in its infancy, Bates noticed how a person could look at a blank wall with no refractive error. Once an eye chart was placed on the wall, however, the person made an effort to see and immediately manifested a refractive error. In the first instance, there was nothing to grab the attention, but in the next instance, the person chased after the letters to try to bring them in clearly.

I'm only speculating, but I believe it was this observation that helped sow the seeds for an array of methods to teach people how to relax their vision: "Fortunately, all persons are able to relax under certain conditions at will. . . . To secure permanent relaxation sometimes requires considerable time and much ingenuity. The same method cannot be used with everyone. The ways in which people strain to see are infinite, and the methods used to relieve the strain must be almost equally varied. Whatever the method that brings most relief, however, the end is always the same, namely relaxation."[28]

Indeed, Bates was quite ingenious in developing various methods to help each person overcome straining and staring. Subsequent Bates instructors over the years have added many other innovative techniques to assist people with diminishing mental strain while simultaneously reestablishing fluid eye movements. That's the beauty of an art—infinite creativity and individuality.

Since mind and muscles mesh with fluid movement, I've chosen to categorize Bates's relaxation techniques based on different types of eye motions: (1) inward activity of the mind's eye; (2) outward activity of the eyes; and (3) combined inward and outward activity of the eyes. Note this is *not* a step-by-step menu process where you do all the activities for the same amount of time and in the same order. "All the methods used . . . are simply different ways of obtaining relaxation," Bates explained.[29] By trial and error, Bates had to find which method would work best for the individual to bring temporary relief from strain. If the method didn't bring immediate relief, he stressed, "It is a mistake to continue the practice of any method which does not yield prompt results. The cause of the failure is strain, and it does no good to continue the strain."[30] The methods are done with prescription lenses removed.

Inward Activity of the Mind's Eye

Inward activity refers to closing your eyelids to shut out the external light and surroundings while using your imagination to keep your eyes in motion, dynamically relaxed. The idea is to rest the eyes by avoiding distracting external stimuli that tempt the stare in the first place. Much like being before a blank wall, there's nothing to chase at with effort. The inward activity—closing the eyes or *palming* (discussed below)—is usually done while sitting comfortably, so it depends on the individual how long it can be done before he or she becomes restless. Some can palm for only a short time, while others can do it for half an hour or more. If done properly, a person should be able to briefly see better than before starting. Some may experience just a flash of clear vision when they first open their eyes, while others may be able to temporarily read a line or two lower on an eye chart.

Closing the Eyes

Simply close the eyes while letting the mind shift from one pleasant thought to another. The blink reflex continues with the eyelids closed, so feel it happen naturally every couple of seconds.

Palming

Some light still gets through the closed eyelids, so palming is done to achieve even more rest. Cup the palms of the hands with the fingers crossed on the forehead in such a way as to avoid contact on the eyeballs. You'll need to get in a comfortable position so that your arms are rested, say on pillow on a table in front of you. With relaxed vision, the field should be black as can be, but make no effort to see it all black at once. In other words, don't stare with your eyes closed. Instead, you mentally shift constantly to keep your eyes mobile. The mental shifting is achieved by using your imagination. It could be shifting from one pleasant thought to another, or it could involve shifting small images in your mind's eye every fraction of a second. Some examples Bates used: imagine seeing a quick succession of black objects (hat, shoe, dress, etc.) one after the other, or if you prefer, a succession of different-colored objects; go through each letter of the alphabet one at time, seeing the letters small and black. The mental shifting is done the entire time while palming. Again, remember to feel the blink reflex.

If you've ever tried meditation, you may notice that palming is somewhat similar. Instead of using a sound as a mantra, you could think of the mantra as a visual image that keeps rhythmically changing. In fact, mentally shifting a small object with the eyes closed achieves such relaxation that a hypnotic state can be induced. Bates was apparently able to perform some eye operations on patients in this state without the use of anesthesia, and many dentists nowadays successfully use a similar hypnotic procedure with their patients.

Sunning is a special form of closed-eye relaxation to help desensitize a person to bright light. With the eyelids closed, face toward the sun and then gently sway (discussed next) and feel the warmth of the sun on the eyelids swing in the opposite direction. This activity can be alternated with palming as well.

Outward Activity of the Eyes

The *outward activities* are meant to be done with the eyes open, but again without wearing glasses or contacts. The purpose of these activities is to incorporate movement to avoid the stare, while at the same time being conscious of fundamentals such as concentric focus and the swing in action.

Swaying

A *sway* is a body movement that has an even beat to it, like a pendulum. The intent is to initiate action that unlocks the stare, permitting the natural reflexive eye movements to take place without strain. You can sway standing up with your whole body, transferring weight from one foot to the other. You can sway sitting down with just your upper body moving from side to side in this tick-tock fashion. If you are in a rocking chair, the rocking motion to and fro is a sway. If you are in an office chair that swivels, the motion is another type of sway. When you turn your head to the left, then to the right, back and forth, back and forth, in a rhythmical manner, this is also a sway.

The types of swaying motions are quite varied. When using the head for sways, you can do the motion horizontally, vertically, forward and backward, or in a circular, rectangular, or elliptical fashion. Contemporary NVI instructors remind people not to fixate when doing the sways; the eyes must have the feeling of *tracing* or *sketching* smoothly in the pattern of the swaying motion.

Regardless of the type of sway, one of the primary purposes is to pay attention to the illusion of the swing. Remember, you don't make the swing happen; it's a reflex. Whatever direction you move, you want to see the apparent movement of stationary objects in the opposite direction of your sway. Probably one of the simplest examples is to stand before a window looking off in the distance. Sway left and right, left and right, and so on. In your peripheral view, you should be able to see the apparent movement of the window frame or a blind swing each way in rhythm. You want to begin to become conscious of this apparent movement so that it becomes an ingrained, unconscious awareness all day long with every action. Bates referred to this illusion as the *universal swing*, as for a person walking along the sidewalk: "The building, the city, the whole world, in fact, may appear to be swinging. . . . So long as he is able to maintain the movement in a direction contrary to the original movement of the eyes, or the movement imagined by the mind, relaxation is maintained."[31]

Although the illusion of the swing is a key element of the sway, another thing you want to realize is concentric focus. A good way to demonstrate the clearer central focus is indoors with two light bulbs or lamps of the same intensity separated by a few feet. Simply sway from one bulb to the other. When your central focus approaches one bulb, it should become brighter, while the one in your peripheral field should get dimmer as it appears to swing away from you.

Shifting

The swaying just mentioned is, in reality, exaggerated shifting. The fluid movement is all a continuum, so there's not really a cutoff point or boundary condition at which the action is distinctly a sway as opposed to a shift. The intent of calling it a sway is to get the illusion of the swing and concentric focus with larger movements so as to gradually, over time, shorten the movements and still see these fundamentals—the stage when shifting can be practiced with letters in a book, on a computer screen, or on a wall chart. For example, shifting may be done from one end of a line of letters to the other end in order to produce apparent movement of the entire row. The whole line of letters should swing in opposition to the shifting. Once this is accomplished, a person may be able to shift from one side of a word to the other to see it swing, then eventually one side of a letter to another to see the letter swing. As with the larger sways, the slighter shifts can be horizontal, vertical, diagonal, circular, or elliptical.

The shifting can also be done from near to far and back again. For example, you might glance at a word in a book and then shift your attention and focus to a number or letter on a calendar or some other type of chart on the wall. If you're beside a window, you can shift from a word or letter at the near point to a small object off in the distance. The illusion of the swing should still be there, although it is more subtle.

Practicing concentric focus is also a good way to help achieve relaxation while shifting. When the text is at a distance just into your blur zone, for example, practice shifting from the top of a letter to the bottom of the same letter. When you briefly look at the top of the letter, it should look more distinctly black than the bottom part of the letter. The bottom part should have the appearance of gray. Then shift to the bottom of the letter and see it distinctly black while the top of the letter becomes gray. Bates describes the benefit:

> The smaller the letter regarded in this way, or the shorter the distance . . . to look away from a letter in order to see the opposite part indistinctly, the greater the relaxation and the better the sight. When it becomes possible to look at the bottom of a letter and see the top worse, or to look at the top and see the bottom worse, it becomes possible to see the letter perfectly black and distinct. At first such vision may come only in flashes. The letter will come out distinctly for a moment and then disappear. But gradually, if the practice is continued, central fixation [concentric focus] will become habitual.[32]

For some people, practicing seeing concentric focus in this way would cause a strain, because they were trying hard to see the center portion black. In such cases, Bates encouraged people not to pay attention to the central portion, but instead, pay attention to the peripheral field being less distinct.

Combined Inward and Outward Activity of the Eyes

These relaxation techniques simply combine the inward and outward activities just described. Bates found that, after relaxing the eyes by closing them or palming for a few minutes, many people would have more success in getting some temporary improvement in their sight. One method is to practice having flashes of clearer vision. Simply close your eyes or palm for a few minutes, then open your eyes for a fraction of a second to glance at a letter a distance away that's normally a bit blurry. Immediately close your eyes and repeat the process. By continually alternating in this manner, you may find that you are able to have clear flashes of the letter. With time and more practice, the clear flashes may become longer and longer. The idea is to ingrain the habit of relaxation so the periods of clear vision are maintained in between blinks.

Other means of alternating activities involve first relaxing the eyes by sitting quietly with the eyes closed or palming for a brief period. Next sway or shift with the eyes open. By alternating this way, many people find it easier to get the illusion of the swing with actual letters and to see one part best in concentric focus.

Some have success by similarly alternating techniques while keeping active. Rather than sitting quietly, they sway or shift with their eyes closed and use their imagination and memory to simultaneously see the swing and concentric focus. Then when they open their eyes, the fundamentals may come easier when swaying and shifting. As Bates said, "All persons, no matter how great their error of refraction, when they shift and swing successfully, correct it partially or completely . . . for at least a fraction of a second. This time may be so short that . . . [one] is not conscious of improved vision; but it is possible for him to *imagine* [emphasis added] it, and then it becomes easier to maintain the relaxation long enough to be conscious of the improved sight."[33]

Here are a few other common Bates techniques using imagination and memory, alternating with eyes closed and open. All these mental images are seen in a continuous swing; trying to see them stationary generates a stare and completely defeats the purpose of relaxation.

- Mentally see a black period swing by shifting from one side of it to the other side, back and forth. The image should be as small as possible but could be any color or any shape, such as round, square, triangular, or irregular. Open the eyes and continue to see the image in this manner.
- Mentally see a black letter O by shifting from one curved side to the other. Imagine the center to be as white as a bright light while shifting. Open the eyes and keep shifting to see the image of the O beaming at you.
- Have small text or a chart at a distance where it is slightly blurred. Close your eyes and imagine one of the letters you know is on the line, such as a *k,* very sharp and black. Use your mind's eye to see it shift slightly to maintain the image. Open your eyes to look at the actual *k* while still imagining it to be black and shifting. Repeat the alternation with eyes open, then closed. Try the same with other letters on the line of text.

SUCCESS STORIES

Meir Schneider is probably the most astounding example of success using Bates's teachings. In his own words, "I was born blind, due to a complication of cataracts (opaqueness of the lens) and glaucoma (excess pressure in the eye). Almost immediately after birth I developed the secondary symptoms of cross-eye and nystagmus (involuntary eye movements)." By age seven, he underwent a number of cataract operations that left 95 percent of the lenses covered in scar tissue. As a result, he could see "only light, shadow and some indistinct shapes. Strong light was extremely painful to my eyes."[34] He was declared legally blind and learned to read Braille.

At age seventeen, Schneider discovered Bates's teachings and started to study and practice them fervently, despite skepticism from most of his family, who thought what he was doing was useless. His grandmother gave him the motivation to continue, for she fully supported and encouraged him from the outset. Meir's vision improvements were slow and gradual, but they were real. Within six months he was able to read text with the aid of very strong glasses. A few months later, the optometrist had to cut the prescription by half. Within a year and half, he was reading print without glasses. He said, "I have never stopped working to improve my vision, and it has never ceased to improve. In 1981, ten years after the whole process began, I was granted an *unrestricted driver's license* [emphasis added] by the State of California."[35]

By curing himself of his blindness, Schneider discovered holistic healing firsthand. His success inspired him to work beyond the eyes. He chose to dedicate his life to studying, teaching, and applying therapy to people with degenerative conditions to help them reawaken their kinesthetic awareness and improve their health. He opened his School for Self-Healing in 1980 and was awarded a Ph.D. in the Healing Arts for his work with muscular dystrophy.

Antonia Orfield's story of improvement differs from Schneider's in that her onset of visual blur at age twelve typified that of many children. Within a couple of years of starting to wear glasses, her prescription for myopia had to be strengthened to compensate for her worsening vision. Her father, concerned that he may have passed on to his daughter his supposedly genetic weak eyes, lent her his book on the Bates Method. After faithfully doing the techniques for three months, her condition stabilized, much to the surprise of her eye doctor. He had confidently predicted further progression of the myopia on her next checkup and further into her teens. It did not progress. In fact, her myopia remained stable for several more years until it once again worsened in her twenties due to new stresses: a whiplash injury and, later, hormonal changes during a pregnancy.

Orfield's interest in vision improvement was rekindled at age thirty-three when she met an optometrist who happened to specialize in myopia reduction. The optometrist was not only familiar with Bates's work but also had improved his own myopia and that of numerous patients. Under his guidance over a period of seven years, Orfield virtually eliminated her significant myopia. She notes the profound impact it had on her at the time: "The whole experience was so fascinating and changed my vision so radically that I decided to become an optometrist."

A former high school English and social studies teacher, Dr. Orfield is now a vision specialist at the Harvard University Health Center. With the instruments she has at her disposal in private practice, she has looked through test lenses equaling her prescription lenses at their strongest stage. She says it now looks like "a swimming blur, the way my father's glasses seemed to me when I was a child. It is hard to believe I spent years looking through them. How was it possible? By gradual, stealthy adaptation. How did I get out of them, then? By gradual de-adaptation."[36]

Another success story is that of Tom Quackenbush, who became one of the world's foremost experts and experienced teachers of Bates vision reeducation after giving up a previous career as an analytical chemist. Quackenbush improved his severe myopia by natural means and has taught hundreds of others how to do the same. Many of his students who once had restricted driver's licenses have since passed the vision test and no longer have the restriction.

Quackenbush studied Bates's extensive writings in depth and concluded that his method had absolutely nothing to do with "eye exercises." Many people have tried in vain to improve their visual acuity by religiously doing eye exercises every day. Not until these people understood the subtle aspects of Bates's principles—typically taught by qualified Bates instructors—and relearned proper, relaxed vision habits did they begin to improve. How the whole notion of eye exercises has grown to completely misrepresent Bates's work is puzzling.

The writer Aldous Huxley also benefited a great deal from NVI. His eyes were damaged by a severe infection at age sixteen, leaving him nearly blind for eighteen months. He depended on Braille for reading and a guide dog for walking during that time. Eventually one eye provided some vision, but with myopia on the order of 20/400. The other eye was capable only of light perception. Twenty-five years later, Huxley learned of the Bates Method and immediately began the techniques. Within two months, he was able to read without his strong prescription glasses. Not only did his acuity begin to improve, but his corneal opacity gradually began to clear up. He noted, "My vision, though very far from normal, is about twice as good as it used to be . . . and the opacity has cleared sufficiently to permit the worse eye, which for years could do no more than distinguish light from darkness, to recognize the ten-foot line on the chart at one foot."[37] Even with this improvement, by his own admission, Huxley still had quite poor vision by normal standards. He wasn't even close to 20/20 acuity. But considering the extent of his blindness before, his improved eyesight was real and significant.

There are even cases of people who have improved their blurred vision naturally with absolutely no knowledge of NVI or the Bates Method. My wife is one such person. When she was in grade seven, her eyes were tested by an optometrist as 20/20 in the left eye and 20/80 (nearsightedness) in the right eye. She was prescribed glasses with a *plano* lens (plain glass) for her good eye and an optical lens to compensate for the worse eye. She couldn't seem to get used to the glasses, so eventually she quit wearing them entirely. Her defiance turned out to be a wise move on her part, because the vision in her right eye eventually restored itself to normal. Bates would have been proud, for, as he stated, "It is fortunate that many people for whom glasses have been prescribed refuse to wear them, thus escaping not only much discomfort but much injury to their eyes."[38]

As an adult, my wife's eyes have been tested by an optometrist at 20/20 acuity, but an intriguing aspect to the story remains. She's now employed as a substitute teacher and occasionally has to work in classrooms with unruly kids. The effort of maintaining order in the classroom sometimes causes her right eye to commence watering. The watering continues for a few hours into the evening, but eventually it subsides with overnight rest and an absence of emotional stress. Interestingly, several articles in Bates's *Better Eyesight* magazine mentioned that excessive eye-watering is a symptom of eyestrain. Relaxation methods that reduce the strain also serve to reduce the copious watering.

Prior to my wife's developing blurred vision, she took weekly swimming lessons for several years as a child. She recalled how, after the day of a swimming lesson, her eyes would be almost glued shut the next morning. It frightened her the first time it happened. She figures she had some type of reaction to the chemicals in the pool that caused an awful yellow sticky mess. It's pure speculation, but did the reaction, similar to the effects of an eye infection, have something do with strain that caused the onset of blur in the one eye? Whatever the cause, the fact remains: her vision restored itself to clarity naturally.

HOW LONG?

Seeing successfully (clearly) again using Bates's techniques requires continual awareness of the fundamentals noted earlier. Don't expect your blurred sight to be dramatically and permanently eliminated, however. To reemphasize: educating your eyes to see clearly is an art form. How quickly a person responds to NVI is highly variable and unpredictable. Certain techniques I mentioned in this chapter have worked for me, and others haven't. You have to find what works best for you.

There will also be relapses along the way. But according to Bates, those who have the best chance for fast and successful improvement are children and those who have worn weak prescriptions for a relatively short period:

> The time required . . . varies greatly with different individuals. . . . It is often necessary to continue . . . for weeks and months. . . . Daily practice of the art of vision is also necessary to prevent those visual lapses to which every eye is liable, no matter how good its sight may ordinarily be. It is true that no system of training will provide an absolute safeguard against such lapses in all circumstances. . . . Generally persons who have never worn glasses are more easily cured than those who have. . . . Persons of all ages have been benefited by this treatment of errors of refraction by relaxation; but children usually, though not invariably, respond much more quickly

than adults. If they are under twelve years of age, or even under six-teen, and have never worn glasses, they are usually cured in a few days, weeks, or months, and always within a year.[39]

The relapses are terribly frustrating, because the rational part of your mind says things like, "This isn't working. This is crazy. Give it up. It's taking too much time and taking too long!" You may have to struggle to rid yourself of such negative self-talk. I've had to many, many times. Patience is more than a virtue with NVI; it's a *must*.

Bates improved his own presbyopia (also called old-age sight) by means of relaxation techniques, and he was frustrated at how long it took him: "My progress . . . was not what could be called rapid. It was six months before I could read the newspapers with any kind of comfort, and a year before I obtained my present accommodative range."[40] He found that about 10 percent of people with presbyopia could improve much more rapidly than he did. The other 90 percent tended to have slow progress too. He was puzzled as to why some cases reversed so quickly, and others did not. He hoped to find the answer, but never did.

David Kiesling has some excellent advice about stages of improvement on his Web site dedicated to the Bates Method:

Improvement isn't linear. When improvement does come, it comes in flashes . . . [and] can happen at any time . . . whenever we let go of the strain to see, and it continues for as long as we don't fall back into strain. One day you might suddenly have a flash of clear vision and not have another for weeks. Or you might have a few most days, and eventually several prolonged periods of clear vision almost every day. The frequency, duration, and quality of clear flashes can be a good indication of how well you're progressing.

At times, you may look at something, see it just as blurry as you used to, and think that you haven't made any progress. That belief itself limits your progress, dragging you into a strained state that ensures a disregard of the progress in relearning to see that you've made up to that point. You already unconsciously learned how to strain in the past, worsening your vision, so don't be disappointed if you keep falling back into those old patterns. All it means is you're straining at the moment. Even people with perfect sight strain now and then, so don't worry about it, as it's nothing that you can't get over.[41]

Aside from extreme fluctuations, from flashes to blur, throughout each day, you will likely experience a less pronounced ebb and flow of visual acuity. To a certain extent, the cause of the fluctuations is out of your control. The continual stresses of life won't magically go away while you're pursuing NVI. Ideally, it would be best if many unnecessary negative stresses could be eliminated or alleviated in conjunction with relaxing the eyesight. But some can't—whether it's the grind in the schoolroom, the office, or the executive boardroom—so you have to adapt to minimize the strain as best you can. You'll be amazed at how your eyes act as a type of barometer to gauge your level of strain under various circumstances. Such fluctuations aren't limited to NVI. It's a fact of the human eye, as noted by Kavner in his practice of behavioral optometry. "Measurements of myopia . . . will sometimes rise as the degree of fretfulness or anxiety increases," he writes. "L. D.'s myopia in her left eye, which was 20/200 when she began therapy, has been testing in the morning of a good day at 20/40; after a tiring day of near-point work, it shoots up to 20/60 or 20/70. And once she is aware that she's not doing well in an examination, she tries all the harder, increasing stress and further reducing acuity."[42]

Like learning any new skill, reacquiring the fundamentals of clear sight feels unnatural at first. Think of it like someone asking you to write your signature with your nondominant hand. It's going to feel awkward, slow, and completely wrong. You'll consciously and unconsciously revert back to old habits of sight time and time again. That's why NVI is no quick-fix solution. Just remember to resist the temptation to "change hands." And besides, once you're well on the road to reducing your blur, you may be pleasantly surprised to find the benefits of eye relaxation aren't just localized. NVI is truly about holistic healing.

6

BALANCE

As it acts in the world, the Tao
is like the bending of a bow.
The top is bent downward;
the bottom is bent up.
It adjusts excess and deficiency
so that there is perfect balance.

LAO TZU[1]

A popular poster depicts an old black-and-white photo of steelworkers on a lunch break from skyscraper construction. Taken in 1932 at the Rockefeller Center in New York City, the snapshot captured the workers sitting side by side on a narrow steel beam suspended from a crane, their feet dangling in the sky. You can tell from the small size of objects in the distance and below that the beam was many stories aboveground. Much like trapeze artists or high-wire performers at the circus who don't bother with a safety net, the workers weren't protected by any special safety gear. Yet they all had a very nonchalant and relaxed appearance. Just another day at the office.

Old newsreels of skyscraper construction in those days filmed the steel erectors darting rapidly like cats with great agility from one beam to another. They displayed no signs of trepidation. An exceptional sense of balance and fearlessness were more than just important skills for getting the job done. Those skills were absolutely critical if the workers wanted to return the next day. One false step, and that was it!

For those with a fear of heights, the usual recommendation is: Whatever you do, don't look down. The intent of the advice is to keep people moving and prevent them from tensing up even further. If they look down, they're apt to stare; a sense of vertigo and panic may then set in, compounding the anxiety they're already experiencing. The next stage might be to stop and hold on with a death grip, refusing to budge an inch, the immobility of staring having translated itself into a total body lock. To prevent a scenario such as this, you have to be calm and "collected." You must "pull yourself together." Don't (figuratively and literally!) "fall to pieces."

Vision plays a significant role in balance. Consequently, it cannot be studied and treated in isolation. If you have blurred vision, your sense of balance is most likely out of whack to a certain degree, since compensations are made elsewhere. Because of your innate adaptability to adjust to stressors, the signs of strain may be completely blocked from your awareness. Even if you do have signals, you're not likely to make any connection with blurred vision and other symptoms.

Little did I realize my NVI journey would go beyond the eyes. Clearing visual blur is a much broader health issue.

BALANCING ACT

Sight, hearing, smell, taste, and touch: those are the five senses as we know them. It seems fairly basic—we see with our eyes, hear with our ears, smell with our nose, taste with our tongue, and touch with our skin. If only it were that simple. In fact, how we consciously perceive stimuli via the senses remains a mysterious and complex matter. Engineering professor and science educator James Calvert notes, "Empirical knowledge of how the senses behave is extensive, but it only describes and does not explain. There seem to be few areas of modern science so important and interesting to us in which the fundamental knowledge is so incomplete. . . . The senses do not interact solely with consciousness, but also with subconscious and involuntary responses to the environment."[2]

Research is finding that humans are able to receive visual data through the other sense channels. A teacher may not have eyes in the back of her head, but she can receive visual information through the senses of taste, touch, and hearing. Sensory augmentation and substitution devices have been developed to help give blind people artificial sight. During laboratory tests, one system that connects to sensory receptors in the tongue "enabled blind people to recognize letters, catch rolling balls, and watch candles flicker for the first time."[3] Another type of system uses sound waves and the sense of hearing to enable blind people to see rudimentary structures, forms, and shapes in their mind's eye.

The symbiotic and synergetic action of the senses is especially noteworthy when it comes to dynamic balance. We sometimes even use the word *sense* to describe balance, for people may speak of their sense of balance being affected. Adept athletes are often described as having excellent hand-eye coordination. So we intuitively know that efficient and effective movement requires muscular coordination and good eyesight.

Actually, balance is primarily dependent on three "systems" of senses: (1) the inner ear (vestibular system); (2) the eyes (vision); and (3) muscle and joint awareness (proprioception). Let's check out the role of each:

Vestibular System

The vestibular system is located in both our ears, so it is considered a dual function with hearing. Also called the inner-ear system, it acts like a gyroscope, sensing the effects of gravity on our center of mass, whether body movements are forward, backward, vertical, horizontal, circular, tilted, or a combination of all these. Even something as basic as walking is highly dependent on proper vestibular functioning.

To appreciate just how important the vestibular system is in our lives, consider a condition such as Ménière's disease, which somehow changes the fluid volumes within a portion of the inner ear. According to the National Institute on Deafness, the disease causes a range of symptoms, "including vertigo or severe dizziness, tinnitus or a roaring sound in the ears, fluctuating hearing loss, and the sensation of pressure or pain in the affected ear. . . . Vertigo, often the most debilitating symptom of Ménière's disease, typically involves a whirling dizziness that forces the sufferer to lie down. Vertigo attacks can lead to severe nausea, vomiting, and sweating and often come with little or no warning."[4] The disease also plays havoc with vision, causing involuntary twitching or bouncing of the eyeballs. Such uncontrolled eye movements make tracking and focusing on objects or print very challenging. Double vision and blurred vision can ensue. Concentration problems, anxiety, and "brain fog" may also be symptoms. In extreme cases, sufferers can be incapacitated at home with symptoms lasting for hours at a time.

Since there is no clear-cut cause for Ménière's disease, researchers are investigating the impact of environmental factors—such as noise pollution and viral infections—as well as biological factors. For less-extreme inner-ear dysfunctions, vestibular problems have many possible causes, including "a variety of infectious, metabolic, toxic, allergic, and physical traumas." With physical traumas, "postconcussion and whip-lash patients frequently complain of such typical inner-ear symptoms as dizziness, loss of balance, slurred speech, headaches, blurred vision, concentration problems, [and] poor memory."[5] What do all the causes have in common? They're all different forms of stress.

When inner-ear disorders are present, a person tends to compensate—in fact, overcompensate—in other ways. Psychiatrist Harold Levinson explains: "When an inner-ear dysfunction results in sensory scrambling or impaired coordination, extra concentration is required to compensate. Individuals with these problems must often devote all their energy and effort to task performance . . . always in a controlled state of high alert—always on guard. But the body pays a price. The need to constantly overconcentrate quickly brings on fatigue and burnout. Many . . . require extraordinary amounts of rest and sleep to recover."[6]

Here we come back to the discussion of staring and concentrating. Once glasses are placed in front of the eyes, you can understand why they do not correct the problem; they only compensate, locking in the staring and overconcentration. Thus, prescription lenses are more appropriately called *compensatory* lenses.

Vision

Vision plays a huge role in balance, because there is much more to vision than simply being able to read or look directly at an object of interest. The function of the eyes in the balancing act is to gather all sorts of information in our external environment to constantly gauge our every move. It's been estimated that we rely on our vision for 80 percent of our sensory input, mostly without being aware of it.

In chapter 5, we discussed the Bates fundamental of concentric focus—the anatomical fact that clearest detail and sharpest color is in the center, with the intensity of focus gradually diminishing in the peripheral field. An inverse relationship is the case for sensing movement with our eyes. The *rods,* which are the movement receptors on the retina, are nonexistent in the center and gradually increase the greater the distance from the center. Their density reaches a peak at midperiphery and then lessens toward the outer periphery. The ratio of peripheral vision to central vision is about ninety-nine to one; so from this whopping difference, it could be argued that the dominant function of our eyes is peripheral—to sense movement.

In addition to peripheral vision, the eyes have another unique ability, to sense the location and orientation of objects beyond the central field of vision. A phenomenon called *blindsight,* which gives the eyes a subliminal type of spatial perception, was first discovered in people who had suffered a head injury. For example, although both eyes might be functioning in a brain-damaged person, the brain damage shuts off sight perception in the right-hand field of vision. Yet such individuals are able to accurately locate objects they cannot see in their blind zone. With incredible accuracy far exceeding chance guessing, they can point to objects, describe either vertical or horizontal orientation of objects, and even detect the direction of moving objects.

These peripheral and subliminal aspects of vision are essentially subconscious and reflexive. Vision is, in fact, largely a reflexive action, which means the eye muscles make all sorts of involuntary movements in response to balance cues. If you quickly turn your head to the left, your eyes first move to the right, then suddenly snap to the left. If you quickly look up, your eyes initially roll down, and then snap up. This pattern of eye movements, called *nystagmus,* happens whether the eyes are open or closed. It's a further indication that seeing is much more than a cognitive skill. Levinson writes, "The eyes automatically react to a change in balance, regardless of whether or not they actually see that change. This suggests that although nystagmus is a visual aid, it is not necessarily vision dependent. Nystagmus is in fact an automatic, reflex response controlled by the human balance center: the inner-ear system. . . . Defects in nystagmus are such a frequent by-product of vestibular dysfunction that they are the most accurate means of diagnosing this dysfunction."[7]

Normal nystagmus has a regular beat—yes, another rhythm. Testing for an inner-ear disorder checks for "abnormal, irregular, or exaggerated nystagmus, or for an absence of nystagmus where it should be present."[8] The tests are best done when the person's eyes are closed, because interestingly, some can actually suppress nystagmus and other eye movements by staring. Some can even suppress the movements when their eyes are closed, simply by concentrating hard. So the ability to compensate by staring and concentrating, skills at which those with visual blur excel, can mask a balance problem.

Vision plays a key role in the intricate balancing act of living. That's why blurred vision or visual disturbances are symptoms of so many diseases and disorders. At least forty-five medical conditions list blurred vision as a symptom.[9] Bates was well aware of the correlation, for he stated, "It is an interesting fact that all diseases of the eyes and all diseases of the body are generally associated with eye tension."[10] The very words *disease* and *disorder* literally mean not at ease and not in order. Blurred vision is one of nature's ways of compensating.

Proprioception

I think of proprioception as our inner sense of touch. Our outer skin detects feelings, pressure, and temperature changes from the external environment. Our internal touch perception is mostly subconscious, but nevertheless present. Deep pressure receptors provide feedback of position and motion in the joints, tendons, and muscles. If we didn't sense where our limbs were in space, where they've just been, or where they're going, it would throw us off kilter.

In addition to the important role of vision, proprioception also plays a dominant role in the balance equation. In the same way sensory input from sight helps direct reflexive eye-muscle movements, proprioceptive sensory input helps direct reflexive muscle movement throughout the rest of the body. Vision and proprioception may be categorized as separate, but they work in harmonious union.

Most people can probably relate to the effects on the inner-ear system if they've had bouts of dizziness or vertigo during the flu or after spinning round while frolicking. It is difficult to imagine, however, what it would be like to be able to move yet be completely devoid of most proprioceptive sensory input. It has happened in very rare cases, and the impact is devastating and debilitating.

Ian Waterman was only nineteen years old when he was stricken seriously ill. He contracted a virus that destroyed specific nerves, leaving him without a sense of touch from the neck down. Although he'd become totally bedridden, the nerves of his motor functions were not affected. He retained the ability to move his muscles, but without the proprioceptive feedback he was, for the most part, very much paralyzed in bed. He desperately wanted to simply sit up on his own but was unable to do so.

Once others put him in a sitting position, he gradually learned how to feed himself again. To clutch a fork, he had to concentrate intently on every motion in his arm, elbow, wrist, and fingers. But to his dismay, while he was managing these motions, his other arm would start to float up on its own and wander in an aimless manner. "Why the hell did it do that? . . . My body had looked after itself before. Why couldn't it now? What was I going to do?" he asked plaintively.[11]

Through trial and error and sheer willpower, Ian eventually managed to get up to a sitting position in bed entirely on his own. This movement, which most take for granted each morning when rising, took a tremendous amount of planning and concentration to achieve. "I was sitting there swaying a bit," he recalled, "but sitting. I relaxed my concentration and allowed myself some congratulatory thoughts and in so doing collapsed back onto the bed."[12] Amazingly, he managed this milestone achievement with the aid of *vision*. As he continued to practice sitting up and relearning other movements, he relied almost entirely on his eyes to guide him. Once he'd lost the peripheral feedback of touch and proprioception, all his motions had to be performed with visual feedback.

After arduous months and years relearning how to move, Ian ultimately walked again without crutches or canes. But the movement wasn't the same as before; it was very stilted and jerky. His world became one of constant anxiety, for if even the slightest thing were to disturb his concentration, it could potentially break his equilibrium, and he would come crashing down. For every movement, he has to watch what he wants to do with intense central focus. As a consequence, his peripheral vision gets blocked:

> I don't wander around looking for flowers. I look for paths. I just have to look at my feet. I lose peripheral things—the aesthetics do suffer. . . . I tell myself, and I think I can believe it, that when I am able to go down to the forest, [once I stop] I take in more than others, because I'm most aware of all the effort involved in my being there. . . . I always have to think where I am and what I'm doing. . . . However beautiful the scene I have to concentrate on what I'm doing, especially on soft ground. Normally if I go anywhere I remember all the little potholes. You might remember a walk for the views. I just remember the walking.[13]

The other price he pays for continual and intense central focus is exhaustion from overconcentration, a compensating action. Not only is Ian's focus and concentrated effort very exhausting, but the intervals between motions are tiring as well. He needs a great deal of muscular tension to stay still. Some animals are able to be rigid as statues between movements, but such stillness for humans is not possible without effort. As biomechanicist Nicholas Bernstein noted, "Mammals find similar locking superfluous, and return to it only in cases of disease. . . . In the norm there is no rest in mammals and human beings. Even the set immobility of a cat or tiger is quite unlike the immobile period in a reptile—it is sufficient to watch its tail."[14] So-called still models for painting have to continually make minor and subtle movements to maintain the appearance of statues.

By closing our eyes and walking, we can get an idea of what it would like to be blind. With the inner-ear system functioning along with proprioception, it's still possible to move with balance. Using aids such as canes or guide dogs, the blind can move along reasonably well, but the movement isn't as fluid as the sighted because of the tension involved. They also rely much more on their hearing as a substitute for environmental clues to movement. But if you were to lose your vision *and* your muscular sense, your balance would be gone, too.

Ian was at a garden party one night where a bonfire and house lights supplied enough ambient light for him to see the ground and his movements in the night environment. Later in the evening, a fireworks display suddenly played havoc with his eyes and immediately thwarted his balance and security. Jonathan Cole, one of his physicians, describes what happened: "The brilliant flashes of light momentarily reversed the dark adaptation of his eyes and blinded him [in between fireworks flashes] for the darker surroundings. He began to falter on his feet and had to tense up. The only way he could continue to enjoy the party was by not looking at the fireworks."[15]

Just as abnormal eye movements are a reliable indicator of a balance problem, the manner in which we walk and move similarly gives accurate clues. Careful observation may point to signs of coordination problems with such symptoms as flat feet, toeing-in or toeing-out, knock-knee, double-jointedness, and scoliosis.

One of the tests used to check a balance problem is called *tandem walking*. As Harold Levinson describes it, this involves "walking a straight line by putting one foot in front of the other in a heel-to-

toe fashion. Poor heel to toe placement, poor foot or leg coordination, swaying, or loss of balance are typical signs of inner-ear dysfunction."[16] There are other types of tests to check balance while standing on one leg. Many may be able to successfully do these tests with their eyes open because they are compensating with visual clues. Once they close their eyes, though, the moment of truth arrives. That's when the difficulties appear. These types of tests accurately diagnose a balance problem in up to 80 percent of cases.*

From this discussion, I hope you can appreciate how the balance trio of the vestibular system, vision, and proprioception is a whole-body process. If one system is off even the slightest, the other two carry more of the burden. Without the modern understanding of this triple play in balance, Bates intuitively made the connection.

BATES ON BALANCE

If you wear glasses and have found that every new pair or change in prescription required a period of adjustment, then you were experiencing the effects of a slight balance disturbance at play. Did you get a bit of dizziness, a headache, and maybe a hint of nausea? Did walking and moving feel a bit weird? When the sight is artificially cleared, the external environment immediately becomes distorted—images appear a different size than normal, they look a modified distance away, colors are dulled, and depth perception is flattened. Even if the distortions are subtle for weaker prescriptions, adjustments and compensations are made elsewhere in the attempt to maintain equilibrium. The initial odd feelings more or less wear off once the adaptation period has set in. But the off-balance effect continues—only it's hidden from awareness for much of the time. Aches and pains eventually show up, an entirely unhealthy response in the long run. Bates describes the process:

---

*Forty years after my classroom vertigo episode and visual disturbances led to prescription glasses, vestibular testing confirmed that I had a previously undiagnosed balance problem. The difficulties with balance under certain tests were immediately manifest when my eyes were closed.

Every oculist knows that patients have to "get used" to [glasses], and that sometimes they never succeed in doing so. . . . The strong concave glasses [for nearsightedness] . . . make all objects seem much smaller than they really are, while convex glasses [for far-sightedness] enlarge them. . . . All glasses contract the field of vision to a greater or less degree. . . . Annoying nervous symptoms, such as dizziness and headache, are sometimes produced. . . . When glasses do not relieve headaches and other nervous symptoms it is assumed to be because they were not properly fitted, and some practitioners and their patients exhibit an astounding degree of patience and perseverance in their joint attempts to arrive at the proper prescription. A patient . . . was fitted sixty times by one specialist alone, and had besides visited many other eye and nerve specialists in this country and in Europe. He was relieved of the [headache] in five minutes by the [relaxation techniques] . . . while his vision, at the same time, became temporarily normal.[17]

Bates's profession and life's work was "focused" on the eyes, but the benefits of NVI extend to whole health. "Tension, besides affecting the eyeball," he wrote, "is also manifest or can be demonstrated in any or in all parts of the body."[18] Bates also wrote about the importance of balance—good posture, especially in the spine, together with efficient muscle movement. He viewed the athletics of the ancient Greeks as a model of efficiency. Their goal, he said, "was to produce a condition in which all the muscles worked harmoniously together and responded instantly to the mind's desire, thus securing a maximum of activity with a minimum expenditure of energy." The lesson to be learned from their athletic pursuits was "such a perfect balancing of the body that whether it is at rest or in motion its centre of gravity is always kept exactly over its base. . . . In this condition there is said to be a complete connection of all the muscles with the centre of gravity. . . . The spine is perfectly straight. . . . Extraordinary precision and beauty of movement results."[19]

When you consider the complex balancing role of the vestibular system, vision, and proprioception, the Bates fundamentals and techniques described in the last chapter should make much more sense. The first time I read about doing swaying movements to get the illusion of the swing, I thought the concept was rather goofy. I couldn't understand why it could possibly help improve vision. Not only do I get it now, but I also think it's truly amazing that Bates did have such a holistic view in his day.

He felt that motion sickness was a signal of strained vision; people so affected felt discomfort from movement seen in the peripheral field. They were consciously or subconsciously attempting the impossible—trying to stop the illusion of oppositional movement. If you strain or stare in planes, boats, or other moving vehicles, you interfere with the reflexive eye movements produced by the inner-ear system, and the strain causes dizziness and nausea.

In 1920, Bates's clinic dealt with a visually impaired man who suffered a number of other concurrent health problems. In particular, he was quite deaf. Bates's assistant, Emily Lierman, had to almost scream into his better ear to make him hear. The man also complained of head noises and drumming in the ears, conditions which would often last for periods of three to ten days. He suffered from severe insomnia, sometimes being up all night. When he did sleep, it was light and fitful, with very wild dreams and nightmares. During the day he also suffered splitting headaches. In addition, Lierman noticed the man walked very clumsily in the clinic, as if intoxicated, bumping into furniture.

After a few months of regular eye-relaxation methods, the man's eyesight improved quite significantly. His other health problems began to abate as well. He reported, "I have been sleeping very much better, the dreams have become much less disturbing, and the headaches have practically ceased."[20] Lierman noted his hearing had improved quite a bit, too; she only had to raise her voice slightly above a conversational tone for him to hear. She also noticed that he was walking almost normally, a far less clumsy gait than when he started. Physicians had previously attributed his clumsy condition as "incipient locomotor ataxia." That's a fancy term for describing an outcome—a loss of muscle control.

Ataxia could have a number of causes. But in this man's case, it was part and parcel of an entire balance disorder.

People who are off-balance may not have any such obvious symptoms. To be unhealthy is to be unbalanced to a certain degree. The signs may be much more subtle and unnoticeable to others. Or you may have signals that you ignore or suppress with palliatives. You need to develop an awareness; tune in and "listen" to what your body is telling you. You'll be amazed how everything is linked, especially with the muscles.

MUSCULAR TENSION

Over 650 muscles throughout the human body are involved in every move we make, whether the movement is initiated consciously while awake, subconsciously while sleeping, or autonomic (involuntary actions of the nervous system such as heartbeat, breathing, and blinking). To initiate such motion, a muscle must strain in response to a stress; it contracts, becoming shorter and wider, while simultaneously tensing up like a guy wire. Muscle contraction is essential for living; it's the natural reaction to the force of gravity. It's a healthy condition in response to eustress. As Alexander Technique teacher Glynn MacDonald explains:

> Muscles . . . are in a state of mild contraction even when seemingly still. Maintaining a static (unmoving) posture demands muscular activity just as any movement does. Just to stand, the muscles which oppose one another on either side of the knee, hip, and ankle must exert an equal and opposite tension. This stabilizes the joints and prevents them from collapsing under the body's weight. Movement is simply the change from one stance to the next. When you move one of your limbs, you increase the state of contraction on one side of the joint and decrease a proportional amount on the other side.[21]

Continuous or excess muscular contraction can eventually lead to distress. Contraction lasts for only so long, as the tension becomes exhausting if held for an extended period. Selye notes, "It seems to be one of the most fundamental laws regulating the activities of complex living beings that no one part of the body must be disproportionately overworked for a long time."[22] Straining to see by squinting and staring is tiring in comparison to the fluid movement of proper refractive rhythm. It's much like standing still in one spot for too long without shuffling or adjusting positions; it becomes very tiring compared to walking for the same period of time. It's not only tiring but also problematic.

A case in point was a soccer team (ironically sponsored by a local optician) of thirteen-year-old boys in England in 1999 who had a terrible record because of their limited movement. At one stage, they lost to opponents by scores of 17–0, 20–0, 23–0, and 25–0. Most of the players were myopic and already wearing glasses. One boy offered his explanation of why his team did so poorly compared to others in the league: "They just pass [the ball] while we're busy standing there or sitting down or whatever."[23] The nearsighted boys were so adept at eye immobility that the habit became ingrained with their whole attitude and posture.

Muscular tension needs to be released with temporary rest until the muscles are called into action again. That's why autonomic movements are rhythmical, constantly alternating between contraction and relaxation. The problem for chronically contracted muscles is the tension tends to linger and leads to rather unusual consequences. Overworked muscles can have residual tension remaining in the form of small contraction knots, called trigger points, in individual muscle fibers. These trigger points lead to all sorts of aches and pains.

Clair Davies had firsthand experience with trigger-point pain, but he didn't know it at the time. Davies had suffered acute and unremitting pain in his shoulder that not only caused insomnia but also threatened to end his work as a piano rebuilder and tuner. He'd made the rounds to various types of specialists, but nobody seemed to understand his shoulder problem, let alone know how to rid him of the pain. He eventually took matters in his own hands—literally. He studied *Myofascial Pain and Dysfunction: The Trigger Point Manual,* by Dr. Janet Travell and Dr. David Simons. They are considered medical pioneers in the study of trigger points. Travell was the U.S. White House physician during the

Kennedy and Johnson administrations, while Simons started his career as an aerospace physician, researching the physical effects of the stress of weightlessness. The two of them contributed many decades of their lives to the research on trigger points and pain.

Davies not only methodically studied Travell and Simons's manual day and night but also began applying self-therapy to the numerous trigger points he'd found. He completely healed his shoulder within a month. It was such a profound experience that Davies, at the age of sixty, decided to abandon his lucrative and prestigious career in the piano business to start over in the massage-therapy business. Now a certified massage therapist, he has written an excellent layperson's guide, *The Trigger Point Therapy Workbook,* which details how to locate trigger points and how to deactivate them. Other noteworthy trigger point manuals are *Pain Erasure,* by Bonnie Prudden, and *Trigger Point Self-Care Manual* and *Trigger Point Therapy For Myofascial Pain,* both by Donna Finando. Prudden and Finando each trained under the tutelage of Dr. Travell.

Common causes of trigger points include the trauma of birth, accidents, illnesses, sports injuries, and the strain of repetitive, overworked motions. These are all forms of stress that cause muscle contraction. Once trigger points develop, muscles begin two bad habits—*splinting* or *substitution*—to avoid the sensation of pain or discomfort. Bonnie Prudden explains:

> Splinting is a shortening of the muscle into spasms in an attempt to guard against pain. Eventually, the shortening of those muscles protecting the body with spasm becomes chronic; the muscles actually lose their ability to relax. . . . Muscles are terrible slaves to habit, and if the habit of splinting is in force long enough, it's very hard to break. The other bad habit [is] substitution. . . . The muscles are hurt, and they cannot move as they were meant to . . . so we substitute other muscles, muscles not designed for that job or not capable of handling two jobs. Then we get into another kind of trouble.[24]

The other type of trouble is developing unnatural motions elsewhere in the body to take over. It becomes a vicious cycle, because splinting and substitution lead to postural changes, trigger points, and pain elsewhere. Splinting and substitution appear to come into play with a very common visual disorder. According to the American Vision Institute, accidents, birth trauma, and poor posture are all known to cause *astigmatism*. This condition is well described in *Improve Your Vision Without Glasses or Contact Lenses* by Stephen Beresford and colleagues:

> Astigmatism is a condition in which the eyeball and/or cornea [outer layer of eye] are warped, distorting and blurring the image on the retina. . . . [The condition] can rapidly change and reverse direction, especially after a neck injury. . . . Patients who suffer whiplash in automobile accidents [often] develop astigmatism within a few hours!
>
> Although astigmatism is usually not genetic in origin, it can result from a difficult birth in which the skull and eyesockets become permanently elongated as the baby is squeezed out. . . . When the head is habitually tilted to one side, usually the result of a bad posture, the extraocular muscles [the muscles attached to the eyeball] adapt by pulling unequally, causing the eyeball and/or cornea to buckle and warp.
>
> Astigmatism is probably the most common visual defect because few people have perfect posture. In most cases, the amount of astigmatism is small and doesn't cause much loss of acuity.[25]

Does the trauma of birth set up trigger points that cause other visual difficulties such as crossed eyes and myopia? It seems very plausible. Toddlers also suffer through many illnesses and viruses as their immune systems develop. They're also prone to falls and minor head injuries. Do these circumstances lead to some preschoolers developing myopia and other visual problems prior to learning how to read and write? I would suspect so.

Then there's the issue of the treatment itself—prescription lenses placed permanently before the eyes, immobilizing the muscles to maintain contraction. It's a well-known fact that splinting and substitution automatically occur when braces, casts, or slings are used to immobilize limbs after injuries such as broken bones, sprains, or dislocations. It only stands to reason that glasses keep the eye muscles chronically tight and never give them a chance to relax, hampering their ability to focus the eye naturally.

Trigger points exert tremendous control; they don't let up easily, since, according to Davies, they "don't respond to positive thinking, biofeedback, meditation, and progressive relaxation. Even physical methods can fail if they're too broadly applied."[26] As well, Davies says, stress and strain play a huge role: "Tension, anxiety, and everyday nervousness can make trigger point therapy ineffective."[27] Perhaps this helps explain why NVI fluctuates so much and is not a quick-fix proposition. There is an ebb and flow to contraction and relaxation of overly tense eye muscles.

BEYOND THE BLUR

The impact of muscle control and excess contraction on health is quite astounding. My health problems went beyond the blur and, as I was to discover, they were all connected.

Before starting NVI, I thought my general health was fairly good for the most part. Through regular exercise and a well-balanced diet, I stayed in good physical condition, maintaining the same weight as in my teenage years. I've also never taken up smoking. Yet a few health issues continually dogged me. One, of course, was my nearsightedness. But there were others. I was a constant mouth breather who caught many severe and lengthy sinus colds every year. Even people who were smokers and physically unfit caught fewer colds that I did. I once had nasal surgery to try to improve my nose breathing and immunity, but to no avail.

Another annoying health issue I dealt with for years was a recurrent stiff neck. Have you ever had this problem? It hurts to turn your head, so you have to do a type of full-body swivel—as if you're in a body cast—to look at something off to the side. I had suffered the problem on and off for years and had no idea what caused it. Because I caught so many head colds, I eventually made the connection that a stiff neck was a precursor to getting a cold. But other times I would have just the stiff neck. In those instances, I figured I'd been sleeping in a contorted position on the pillow the night before. What was puzzling was that the stiff neck would usually get *worse* as the day went on, not better. I would have expected the opposite to occur.

When I played the piano as a boy, I spent long hours of practice hunched over, intently reading the music closely through glasses while concentrating hard not to make mistakes. I would frequently get a pain in my left shoulder-blade area. At the time I assumed it was caused by not having any back support as I sat on the piano bench. It soon became a routine during every practice to reach back and rub beside my shoulder blade to try to relieve the discomfort.

Blurred vision, nose-breathing problems, poor immunity to resist severe sinus colds, stiff neck, pain in the shoulder-blade area. The attitude I took was essentially acceptance; everyone has health issues, and mine weren't a big deal in the major scheme of things. A lot of people had far more serious health problems with which to contend.

Soon after I commenced my NVI program, I began to take note of some subtle changes. I first noticed that my eyes started to look brighter and healthier. But changes went beyond the eyes. I also noticed muscles in my cheeks and jaw areas seemed to be looser. There was a tingling and numbing sensation, as if they'd been somewhat atrophied and were starting to come back to life again. I could also tap those areas of my face and feel sensations around the eyes.

When I practiced eye relaxation sways and swings, I would sometimes notice twitching in my nose and sinuses. When a clear flash would come on, my eyes would start to water, and I would occasionally have to sneeze at the same time. One night while watching TV, I had a fleeting moment of sharp pain in the left shoulder-blade area while my left eye twitched and began to tear during a flash. The feeling immediately reminded me of the piano lessons.

The next body change I noticed was not so subtle; it was intense. I didn't know what a *really* stiff and painful neck was until this point. One day I had the condition worse than ever. A sharp pain not only emanated from beside my left shoulder blade and up my neck but this time pain extended around front to my chest area, too. It was impossible to sleep that night for two reasons: every time I moved even an inch, I would wince from the jolt of pain in the neck and shoulder; and I was frightened. Could I be having signs of heart trouble? Although I was in good physical condition, I began to panic as my mind raced. I thought my vision health was going to be the least of my problems at that point. I decided I'd better get to the hospital to make sure it wasn't a heart problem.

There I was in the wee hours of the morning at the emergency ward, hooked up to wires and monitored by instruments. The hospital staff couldn't find anything wrong. In fact, the doctor commented on my excellent low resting heart rate and wondered what I did for exercise. He had no explanation for what could be causing the pains. The only advice was to check with my family physician if it didn't improve, so I headed home. At that point, a light bulb clicked on. Right then and there, I was convinced beyond a shadow of a doubt that these symptoms were related to my NVI program.

The aches and pains I was experiencing were a positive sign of health restoration. My body was gradually rebalancing and readjusting as muscular tension released and posture was restored. All three balance systems—the vestibular system, vision, and proprioception—were affected holistically.

REBALANCING

The seemingly unconnected symptoms I'd been experiencing are called *referred pains*. Trigger points, the muscular contraction knots in overly tense muscles, cause pain and other symptoms that mysteriously pop up in zones sometimes far removed from the points themselves. The concept of referred pain is not clearly understood, but the referrals have been well documented from a wealth of case studies. Some of the trigger-point culprits in Davies's shoulder case were located in certain neck muscles. It turns out that muscles in the neck, face, and head can cause a tremendous number of surprising and disturbing symptoms at other locations, as Davies noted:

> Trigger points cause an astonishing variety of symptoms in the head and neck region. Some of the effects they can have may contradict a lot of what you've always believed. Trigger points are known to cause pain and hypersensitivity in your teeth, pain and stuffiness in your ears, pain and redness in your eyes, sinus pain and drainage, stiff neck, chronic cough, and sore throat. Trigger points can cause dizziness and balance problems. They can blur your vision and make the words dance around on the page when you're trying to read. They can make your lips numb, your tongue hurt, or an eyelid droop.
>
> Furthermore, trigger points are responsible for much of the pain associated with temporomandibular joint (TMJ) syndrome and are involved in important ways with the other symptoms of this disturbing condition, including popping and clicking in the jaw, dislocation of the jaw, restriction of jaw opening, and faulty closure of the teeth.
>
> If this isn't enough, Travell and Simons' work has shown that trigger points are often the hidden and unsuspected cause of most headaches.[28]

Many muscles develop trigger points that have a direct impact on vision. The following is a sampling of muscles that, if trigger points are present, can cause blurring of vision or other visual or eye disturbances. In parentheses I indicate the approximate location of the muscle:

- Sternocleidomastoid (front side of neck);
- Temporalis (temple);
- Splenius cervicis (back of neck and skull);
- Masseter (jaw);
- Suboccipitalis (base of skull at back of head);
- Occipitalis (back of head);
- Orbicularis oculi (around the eye); and
- Trapezius (upper back).

The TMJ syndrome Davies mentions is also called a TMJ disorder, a misaligned-jaw condition. Its varied symptoms include headaches; face, neck, and shoulder pain; sinus pains; dizziness; and *blurred vision* and *chest pains*. Amazingly, many people suffer visual blur or visual disturbances because of a problem with the TMJ. Even more coincidental is the link with chest pains that I had experienced.

Dr. Ira Klemons, an internationally recognized expert in the field of TMJ disorders, headaches, and facial pain, has successfully treated sufferers for over thirty years. Over the course of his practice, he discovered that approximately one sixth of his patients had a chest-pain problem. "Many had been to cardiologists and most had been to their physicians or to hospital emergency rooms," he wrote. "Yet in almost every case that we saw, a specific cause for the pain could not be found." The chest pains resolved for 90 percent of those treated for head and facial pain.[29]

Major causes or contributing factors of a TMJ disorder are malocclusion (an improper dental bite or misaligned teeth) and poor dental work. Interestingly, vision research has shown a strong correlation between myopia and both malocclusion and tooth decay.[30] I had several fillings and a couple of extractions as a boy, but who knows whether the work done at the time was poor or not. I also have malocclusion and once had oral surgery to remove impacted lower wisdom teeth. Two dentists recently confirmed that I should have probably had orthodontic treatment as a child, for I now have an "open" bite with very few teeth making contact. Because of my jaw imbalance, malocclusion and accompanying symptoms, they've confirmed I have TMJ disorder.

A couple of years after my heart scare, I began to notice discomfort in my calf muscles when walking. Since I hadn't been doing any different or unusual activities to bring this on, I thought it was odd. But an intuitive idea immediately popped into my head. Was my whole sense of balance previously off enough when I wore glasses that I used to walk with strain, too? My shoes always had strange wear and scuff marks from striking one another when I walked. One shoe would somehow make contact with the other with each stride, yet I was never consciously aware that I was doing it. The telltale marks were there on every pair of shoes I ever owned.

A few days after the onset of leg discomfort, I woke up one morning with severe and painful cramps in my calves. I had to rub them vigorously to release the pain. Because of what I had thought previously when walking, I told my wife it was probably another sign of body tension releasing in conjunction with my improving eyesight. She could appreciate the connection with tension from the shoulders up, yet she thought I was off my rocker this time. But lo and behold, I later found out my hunch was right. In Meir Schneider's *Handbook of Self-Healing* was the following passage: "Without even looking at the body of a nearsighted person, one can predict confidently that he or she will have pronounced tension in the forehead, jaw, neck, shoulders, upper arms and lower back, and *often the calves as well* [emphasis added]."[31] Years earlier, an elderly librarian who had a strong interest in and knowledge of natural health, especially massage and movement, told Schneider, "The calf muscles are connected to vision."[32]

A TMJ disorder is but one of many health problems that can cause dizziness. Ear problems are another big culprit. People with inner-ear difficulties suffer such symptoms as vertigo, nausea, and blurred vision. Recall from the introduction that my first memory in the classroom before getting glasses prescribed was extreme dizziness. Technically, what I had that day was *vertigo*. First there was an immediate visual sensation that the front of the room and blackboard rapidly moved away from me, and the sense of perspective was that it was instantly double or triple the distance away that it really was. Then the spinning of the room started and wouldn't stop. I broke out into a sweat and was queasy.

Did I have a condition that was rooted in the eyes and caused symptoms elsewhere, or did the problem emanate from either the jaw joint or the inner ear and spread symptoms from there? Does one go to an eye doctor, a dentist, an ear doctor, or a physiologist? It becomes an endless chicken-and-egg situation if you consider it in this divided manner. With other health concerns, countless numbers bounce from one specialist to another, never getting satisfactory answers or solutions. People can go for years either being misdiagnosed or being selectively treated in only one area of the body. Health simply cannot be viewed in this piecemeal context for strain-related problems. Rebalancing as part of NVI is definitely a head-to-toe proposition. When you're without undue tension, Janet Goodrich has stated, "you will see with your whole body."[33]

RELEASING BODY TENSION

Dr. Alexander Lowen, founder of the mind-body therapy called *bioenergetics,* noted in 1964, "In my opinion myopia is a functional eye disorder that has become structured in the body as a distortion of the eyeball. It does not differ from other bodily distortions that are the result of chronic muscular tensions. . . . One of the difficulties in working with the myopic eyes is that the tense ocular muscles are not accessible to palpation and pressure."[34] That's the bad news. The good news is that other muscles in the body related to eye tension are accessible to therapy.

As an adjunct to my NVI program, I started to get massage therapy treatments for muscle relaxation of my neck and shoulder areas. The therapist, using a technique called myofascial release, would sense areas of tightness in the connective muscle tissue (the fascia that covers the whole body) to gradually guide the relaxation of tension. The first major release occurred when a spot just under my chin was triggered near the jaw line. The sense of spatial disorientation was immediate and overpowering. If I'd been standing up, I'm sure I would have fallen from the bizarre sensation. During another session, there was a huge release of tension at my left ear.

After those initial sessions, rebalancing aches and pains eventually began to pop up in other areas of my body, including the calf muscles, as noted earlier, as my vision improved. I never thought the NVI process would spread beyond my head and neck; once it became apparent that postural rebalancing was occurring throughout the whole body, however, the massage treatments began to include my feet, legs, hips, and torso. This was accomplished with craniosacral therapy (CST), the gentle technique developed by Dr. John Upledger, an osteopathic physician. The goal of the CST sessions was to help spread the muscle fascia, thereby improving functioning of the central nervous system via the spinal network, from the sacrum (tailbone) to the cranium (skull).

Self-administered trigger-point therapy has also been beneficial. Thanks to Davies's tips, I've managed to target specific muscles that flare up from time to time and apply the deactivation techniques. I have located and deactivated trigger points in many of the muscles previously noted that are known to affect the eyes. The CST treatments also had a way of activating dormant trigger points. By far the most sensitive and painful trigger points have been in my midback (erector spinae) and shoulder blade (rhomboid) on the left side. (The massage therapist joked that the muscles were like guitar strings, so tight that a tune could be played!) Deactivating these trigger points caused sensations to shoot into my jaw, ears, and eyes that felt like an electrifying jolt. I felt a similar sensation when deactivating certain trigger points in my legs. Referred reactions certainly are a strange phenomenon.

Other therapeutic body-work methods include such practices as chiropractic, Rolfing (structural integration), shiatsu, acupressure, and the Feldenkrais Method. The very essence of the Feldenkrais Method is a somatic education to help people tune into their body movements to reestablish motions that have been forgotten or have been habitually incorrect for years. Many have eliminated aches and pains by improving the efficiency of neck, back, and shoulder movements. In fact, Jack Heggie combined Feldenkrais principles with the Bates Method in a program appropriately called Total Body Vision.

In chapter 4, I briefly commented on the work of F. M. Alexander. The Alexander Technique was initially developed for those in the performing arts, but its benefits quickly spread to anyone suffering persistent problems due to muscular strain. Although the method is not considered a medical practice or healing art per se, it can reap significant health benefits. Bates knew of Alexander's accomplishments and praised his work in a 1927 *Better Eyesight* article entitled "Tension":

We may have cases of eye diseases in which it is difficult to relieve the tension, but it may be easy to relieve the tension in the muscles of the stomach or in the various groups of muscles in the arm, or hand, and when such tension is relieved, that of the eye muscles is relieved. . . . A man, by the name of F. M. Alexander, of London, England, has accomplished a great deal in the cure of all kinds of diseases. He says that all diseases of the body are caused by tension. They can all be cured by the relaxation of the tension. . . . It has been a great shock to many orthodox physicians to observe the cures that Alexander has made.[35]

Glynn MacDonald describes the Alexander Technique as "a method for organizing your sensations of movement, both where you are in space and in time, by becoming more conscious of your internal and external world." It is a system of mind and body awareness with three important principles: (1) "the way we 'use' ourselves (move, think, etc.) affects how well we function"; (2) "the organism functions as a whole"; and (3) "the relationship between the head, neck, and back has a paramount influence on the whole organism, its posture and health."[36]

Many NVI students have benefited from studying and applying the Alexander Technique to their program. Peter Grunwald, who is now an NVI instructor and author, significantly reduced his myopia through a combination of the Bates Method and the Alexander Technique.[37] Antonia Orfield, the former teacher turned optometrist, whose success story on myopia reduction was discussed in chapter 5, undertook Alexander Technique lessons. She says: "Alexander teachers do find that vision improves as patients continue lessons and often lens prescriptions need to be reduced or further postural improvement is impossible. . . . I know from experience that posture and vision are interactive. Neck tension is one of the major things that was released with Alexander Technique. Getting my neck 'free and back' and my 'energy up' reduced the amount of lens power that I needed to see clearly and reducing lenses, in turn, further reduced my neck tension."[38]

The first book I had on the Bates Method spoke of tight neck muscles for those who had blurred vision. Since the book incorporated naturopathy, some neck-flexibility exercises were suggested. I did them for a while, but I didn't think they were having any effect on my vision, so I eventually stopped doing them. Even though I'd had a stiff neck from time to time in the past, I thought I had reasonably good mobility with neck rotations and movement when I began NVI. Thus, I prematurely ruled out the impact of the neck. Via nerve sensations and symptoms, our body tells us loud and clear that there is an imbalance. Not paying heed to the cause leads to compensations in movement that eventually start to feel normal and ultimately block out the initial sensations. MacDonald notes, "Alexander showed that it is possible to be unaware of what we are doing [wrong]. It is generally assumed that feelings give us accurate information about our body. When this feedback is incorrect, our sensory appreciation becomes unreliable."[39] The vestibular testing I had done confirmed I didn't have the neck mobility I thought I had. The therapist's cervical findings noted "significant stiffness bilaterally" of side neck flexions as well as "stiffness and decreased stability of the [left] shoulder girdle" due to myofascial restriction.

The various bodywork and postural-improvement techniques I have mentioned all approach the problem from slightly different angles. They share a common link, however, with respect to the importance of proper head and neck movement. Neurology confirms that the neck contains the highest density of nerve receptors for proprioception. Notes Cole, "Both the eyes and the balance organ in the ear require the head to be stable to function."[40] The head must be *dynamically* stable, not constricted in mobility or off-kilter.

Muscles in the face and around the eyes can also benefit from massage, indirectly aiding in the relaxation of tense eye-focusing muscles. Palming, as discussed in the last chapter, seems to provide this type of self-massage as a secondary outcome. The warmth and softness of the touch on the orbicularis oculi muscle surrounding the eye has the therapeutic effect of relaxing that muscle. Meir Schneider, a proponent of massaging muscles in the face and the neck in conjunction with improving vision, states, "One of the most important functions of palming is, in fact, relaxation of the muscles around the eyes."[41]

Most NVI instructors and Bates teachers tend to agree on the importance of proper diaphragmatic breathing (belly breathing) in helping reduce muscular tension. It's particularly important to be aware of shallow-breathing patterns that may take over during times of stress. If you can maintain the habit of proper belly-breathing, the long-term health benefits from such poise will pay off. Yogic breathing techniques (known as *pranayama*) that alternate one nostril closed and one open in harmony with inhalation and exhalation are also known to be helpful for those on an NVI program.

Don't be surprised if other outcomes occur with the removal of muscle tension. The improvement in my vision has coincided with a significant change in my immunity against colds. I once went over three years without catching a head cold or sinus cold. (You're darn right I was keeping track!) I'm no longer a mouth breather, so I believe the reduced body tension together with proper breathing through the nose has dramatically improved my immunity. David Kiesling, whose *Imagination Blindness* Web site is dedicated to the Bates Method, says he was "anosmic (unable to smell) my whole life but recently started sensing certain smells. Thinking is more effortless. I'm more relaxed in general. I rarely get sick anymore. It goes on and on. I've changed my whole approach to everything, and I'm still in the process of doing so."[42]

The imprint of strain throughout your body is as individual as your fingerprints. Two people with blurred vision may have exactly the same lens prescription, but their muscular and postural imbalances could vary considerably. Although there may be some similar tension patterns and symptoms, especially in the neck and shoulders, the release of muscular tension and eye tension through bodywork practices is unique for each person. You have to determine what feels right for you.

HOLISM

Bates concluded that good vision was equated with good health. He made the following comments in the context of concentric focus, but they apply in general to clear sight:

> Since central fixation [concentric focus] is impossible without mental control, central fixation of the eye means central fixation of the

mind. It means, therefore, health in all parts of the body, for all the operations of the physical mechanism depend upon the mind. Not only the sight, but all the other senses—touch, taste, hearing and smell—are benefited by central fixation. All the vital processes—digestion, assimilation, elimination, etc.—are improved by it. The symptoms of functional and organic diseases are relieved. The efficiency of the mind is enormously increased. The benefits of central fixation already observed are, in short, so great that the subject merits further investigation.[43]

Outlandish claims? Only if you assume NVI is being touted as some sort of panacea. But I don't believe that's what Bates was suggesting, even though he documented numerous case studies in which people using his method found improvement in the functioning of the other senses, particularly hearing, as well as improvement in vital processes or relief of symptoms of other disorders. I believe his statements about the general health benefits relate to eliminating mental stress and strain. The subject matter has been further investigated extensively, starting with the work of Selye and growing into a huge field of health research. The results of that research affirm what Bates was suggesting about health as a whole improving with the removal of strain.

If you take the holistic perspective to NVI, then everything fits. The general adaptation to strain is the common denominator with health symptoms beyond the eyes. It's like standing on a trampoline. No matter where you place yourself, there are stresses and strains everywhere due to your body weight. If your weight was off to the side, the distribution would be unbalanced. If the trampoline could speak, it would complain about tightness and reactions in the fabric, springs, and support legs.

But healing extends beyond whole-body physical rebalancing. When we have things "weighing" on our minds, either consciously or subconsciously, the reactions from head to toe are much like an unbalanced load on the trampoline. The role of the mind and emotions is significant in helping fully restore a healthy balance. Let's explore these concepts more in chapter 7.

7

WHOLENESS

These things from ancient times arise from one:
The sky is whole and clear.
The earth is whole and firm.
The spirit is whole and strong.
The valley is whole and full.
The ten thousand things are whole and alive.

Carrying body and soul and embracing the one,
Can you avoid separation?

LAO TZU[1]

Hippocrates said in 202 BCE, "Let no one persuade you to cure the headache until he has first given you his soul to be cured. For this is the great error of our day in the treatment of the human body, that physicians separate the soul from the body."[2] If our eyes are "windows of the soul," then orthodox vision treatment considers only the pane and cuts off the underlying and expansive soul.

This same error of separation is often made by newcomers to NVI. Depending on the source, the Bates Method can occasionally be watered down and misinterpreted as strictly physical therapy: do some eye exercises, and you can whip them back into shape for clearer sight. Many people have committed to such a regimen of eye aerobics only to be disappointed with little to no improvement over an extended period. If a naysayer chuckles with told-you-so glee, a person may be apt to give up, believing NVI is of very little benefit for all the effort.

Some were not deterred by the limitations of a purely physical approach. They knew there had to be more to NVI than what appeared on the surface. They partook in whole-body therapies, as discussed in the last chapter. They also chose to get to the heart of the matter—literally and figuratively—venturing into deep inner realms and emotional healing. Once on that path, their eyesight dramatically improved. A number of these people went on to become NVI practitioners themselves. Although they may all appear as different offshoots of the Bates Method, they share a common thread. As vision therapist John Selby stated, visual recovery is "a deep spiritual restructuring of who you are in the world."[3]

Successful NVI is, indeed, a soul journey. It requires a spiritual conviction affirming not only that there's more to life than meets the eye but that the hidden and mysterious "more" also meets the eye. The rich inner realm profoundly affects the manner in which the eye responds to stimuli and influences health as a whole. Vision healing goes deeper than the physical eyes and optic nerves; its roots extend well into the layers of the mind. Holistic is largely *soul*-istic.

THE MIND

What exactly do we mean by the term *mind*? The scientific explanation seems to suggest that the mind is localized solely inside the head, with the brain simply acting as a central processing unit—a human computer, albeit a supercomputer. The neurological firings and brain waves are somehow by-products of our biochemical body processes. This sort of concept seems to be far too narrow in scope, as there are situations that totally baffle science and call in question the entire notion of the mind-in-the-brain.

A Canadian TV documentary many years ago featured an elderly woman who took care of her adult son. The son was blind, mute, and incapable of learning under conventional schooling. He was thought to be completely disabled mentally. One day when her son was a boy, however, the mother heard some beautiful piano music coming from another room in the house. She assumed it was the TV or the radio. But when she came into the room where the piano was, she found her son playing complex classical music. He hadn't been taught anything, let alone to read sheet music, because of his blindness. Yet there he was playing effortlessly and flawlessly! It was a very moving story.

The son was classified as a *savant*. Dustin Hoffman played the role of a mathematically gifted savant in the popular movie *Rain Man*. The movie was inspired by the true story of Kim Peek, an autistic savant who is a genius in over a dozen subjects but is mentally disabled for the most basic tasks, such as dressing himself. He can recall the more than seventy-six hundred books he's read and has the ability to speed-read at the rate of up to twenty thousand words per minute with 98 percent comprehension. He accomplishes this feat by simultaneously reading the left page with his left eye and the right page with his right eye.

Back during the Civil War era, there was a popular savant who was musically gifted. Mark Twain first encountered him on a train ride and, not knowing who he was, was extremely annoyed at his strange and seemingly barbaric antics. The man constantly swayed violently back and forth in his seat and mimicked the "the hiss and clatter of the train, in the most savagely excited way." He made all sorts of strange sounds for over three hours, and when he did speak, "it was excitedly to himself, in an idiotic way and incoherently." Twain wondered who the man was and where he was headed. The other passengers told him it was Blind Tom, the celebrated pianist. Later Twain attended one of his performances:

When anybody else [a volunteer] plays [the piano], the music so crazes him [Blind Tom] with delight that he can only find relief in uplifting a leg, depressing his head half way to the floor and jumping around on one foot so fast that it almost amounts to spinning— and he claps his hands all the while, too. His head misses the piano about an inch or an inch and a half every time he comes around, but some astonishing instinct keeps him forever from hitting it. It must be instinct, because he cannot see, and he must surely grow too dizzy with his spinning to be able to measure distances and know where he is going to and whither he is drifting. And when the volunteer is done, Tom stops spinning, sits down and plays the piece over, exactly as the volunteer had played it, and puts in all the slips, mistakes, discords, corrections, and everything just where they occurred in the original performance! He will exactly reproduce the piece, no matter how fast it was played or how slow, or whether he ever heard it before or not.[4]

Humility and simplicity are core Taoist values. Compare Twain's description of the savant to these verses from Lao Tzu's Tao Te Ching:

> *Other people have what they need;*
> *I alone possess nothing.*
> *I alone drift about,*
> *like someone without a home.*
> *I am like an idiot, my mind is so empty.*
>
> *Other people are bright;*
> *I alone am dark.*
> *Other people are sharp;*
> *I alone am dull.*
> *Other people have a purpose;*
> *I alone don't know.*
> *I drift like a wave on the ocean,*
> *I blow as aimless as the wind.*[5]

Another enigma to medical science is hydrocephalic disorder. People with hydrocephalus are born without the full brain considered absolutely essential for day-to-day functioning, intelligence, and learning. The condition, in which the cranium is filled mainly with cerebrospinal fluid, is usually fatal within the first few months of birth. Should a child survive, a severe disability is the typical prognosis. But there are exceptions—very remarkable exceptions.

Dr. John Lorber, a British neurologist, gave an account of one such person with hydrocephalus in 1980.[6] A university student with an IQ of 126, who had obtained first-class honors in mathematics and was socially normal, underwent a routine medical examination. The doctor noted that the student's head size was larger than average, so he referred him to Lorber for a brain scan. The scan revealed a thin layer of mantle—a millimeter or so—instead of the normal tissue thickness of 45 millimeters in that region. The student had been living successfully with virtually no brain, yet the condition had gone completely undetected before. His case, although shocking and rare, was nothing new; medical history apparently contains scores of similar such cases, many which had gone undiagnosed until autopsies were performed.

Other mysteries reported in the annals of medical literature defy conventional theories and logical reasoning. There are cases of amputees who report feelings of pain, sensation, and movement in their missing limbs, a phenomenon known as phantom limb. The feelings aren't at the point of amputation, but rather at their missing extremities, such as toes and fingers. There are also now many medically documented cases of heart-transplant patients who feel emotions and have dreams of events that occurred in the deceased *donor's* life. The transplant patients also acquire unusual tastes and cravings for foods they never liked before, foods that were favorites of the donor. Admittedly, these phenomena border on the mystical and spooky, but they do radically shake the conventional Western model of the mind.

The predominant materialistic view is that human existence is all physical "reality," whereby our affective and intellectual characteristics are localized brain functions. For example, the scientific community developed the "triune brain" theory in the 1950s. This theory suggests there are actually three brains in one: the reptilian, or R-system, the limbic, and the neocortex.[7] The R-system corresponds to core body sensory and motor functions necessary for sleep/wake cycles and basic survival.

The limbic brain is supposedly responsible for our vast array of emotions, dreams, memories, and intuitions. The neocortex, considered the highest evolutionary brain, provides us with intellect, logical reasoning, creative thinking, and language.

Contrast this evolutionary, material model with Rudolf Steiner's three-fold view of human beings. In 1910 Steiner, the renowned philosopher and spiritual scientist, described our three-fold aspect as an ascending succession of body, soul, and spirit. The lowest level, the body, develops a physical form from natural mineral substances, grows and reproduces, and perceives the external world via sense organs. These bodily attributes are related to the mineral, plant, and animal kingdoms. The second level of humans, the soul, refers to the unique inner impressions, feelings, drives, and passions we experience based upon our sense perceptions. This second aspect is also evident in animals. The highest level, the spirit, refers to thinking—how we reflect upon our experiences and are guided by right thoughts. This spirit aspect is recognizable in animals to a certain degree, but as a rudimentary type of consciousness.

In this three-fold view of human existence, the soul interpenetrates between the physical and spiritual realms, receiving sensations from "below" and intuitions from "above." The soul is nourished and enriched by both at a very personal, internal level. Steiner suggested that this "intrinsic privateness" of the soul—for example, one may look at the same physical objects that others see, but one cannot perceive or know others' personal sensations—is beyond a simple brain function. "Once we are quite clear about this, we will stop looking at inner experiences as mere brain processes or something of that sort."[8] On the other hand, he noted how the spirit is associated with the brain:

> The whole human body is built up in such a way that the brain, the organ of the spirit, is its crowning glory. We can understand the structure of the human brain only when we look at it in relationship to its function, which is to serve as the bodily basis for the thinking spirit. This is demonstrated by a comparative survey of the animal

kingdom: In amphibians the brain is relatively small in proportion to the spinal cord, in mammals it is larger, and in humans it is largest of all in proportion to the rest of the body.[9]

Spiritual thinking transcends the utilitarian concerns of our material world. It is the pursuit of higher knowledge, the quest for the Divine, awakening the "eye of the spirit" to reveal eternal truths. It is anything but cold and calculating logic that deadens feelings and emotions. On the contrary, Steiner emphasized, "No feeling and no enthusiasm on earth can compare with the sensations of warmth, beauty and exaltation that are enkindled by pure, crystal-clear thoughts relating to higher worlds."[10]

Several Eastern and ancient esoteric traditions have long considered the mind to be nonlocalized. They also believe in different mind dimensions, whereby humans consist of a physical body in combination with a number of "mind bodies." Those with deep intuitive abilities, seers, are said to be able to perceive these subtle bodies. Whatever the role of the brain, the mind (or minds) is a complex holistic interplay that I like to view as tapping into the higher consciousness of the Tao.

UNITY

The error of separation between mind and body is very much a given in our technological era. In fact, the assumptions we make about the mind and body are culturally programmed. Psychologist Ellen J. Langer explains: "From earliest childhood we learn to see mind and body as separate and unquestioningly to regard the body as more important. . . . If something is wrong with our bodies we go to one kind of doctor, while with a 'mental problem' we go to another. Long before we have any reason to question it, the split is ingrained into us in endless ways. It is one of our strongest mindsets, a dangerous premature cognitive commitment."[11]

Ironically, even when discussing the unhealthy split, the pull is so great that the danger even sounds lopsided, with language such as "mindset" and "cognitive commitment." Sigmund Freud, the founder of psychoanalysis, probably played a predominant role in influencing and perpetuating this notion of a split. The *psyche,* or the mind, was considered an entity to be studied, coded, and deciphered separately from the body. He once predicted, however, that a link would someday be found between the mind and body, what he called, in technical terms, *somatic compliance.*[12]

Taoists weren't prone to the error of separation, for they knew the unity of mind and body. Consider the following passage:

> *Thirty spokes join in the wheel's hub;*
> *the center hole makes the wheel useful.*
> *Mold clay into a pot;*
> *the space within makes the pot useful.*
> *Build doors and windows for a room;*
> *the cut openings make it useful.*
> *Therefore being is for benefit,*
> *Nonbeing is for usefulness.*[13]

The human body (being) is a form of matter that works in seamless harmony with the mind (nonbeing). By tapping the immense hidden power and usefulness of the mind, we benefit with body actions.

Not all medical science separates being and nonbeing. Psychosomatic medicine is a specialty field that studies how the mind and body interact to cause puzzling diseases or disorders. People with a psychosomatic condition can sometimes complain of ailments and symptoms that are very real to them. Yet doctors are unable to diagnose any organic cause for the condition—in other words, there is no physical evidence of a faulty "part" in the system.

There are also cases where known physical conditions can be reversed with the power of mental suggestion. An example is people who have warts. In several studies, patients were able to successfully rid themselves of warts under hypnosis. In one study, the patients were asked to be more selective with their curing. By using only the power of their hypnotized minds they were able to successfully remove the warts on just one side of their bodies![14]

The placebo effect continues to be one of the biggest medical enigmas. It's more the power of belief than the power of suggestion. Patients have a strong conviction that a special drug or treatment is being administered when, in actuality, they aren't receiving anything of medicinal value. They simply take a fake pill and look at the doctor's white coat, and healing eventually takes place. Dr. Albert Schweitzer explained that the "witch doctor succeeds for the same reason all the rest of us [medical doctors] succeed. Each patient carries his own doctor inside him. They come to us not knowing that truth. We are at our best when we give the doctor who resides within each patient a chance to go to work."[15]

The placebo effect not only heals but has been known to cause adverse side effects. Consider the surprising result during a clinical trial for a new cancer drug: "Hidden in the background . . . of a 1983 *World Journal of Surgery* article on a chemotherapy trial for gastric cancer, buried as a single numerical entry in a single chart, is a fascinating notation: Nearly one-third of a control group—a group that received only a salt-water placebo in place of powerful chemicals—had experienced 'alopecia.' Alopecia—mirror-avoiding, clumps-on-the-pillow-every-morning hair loss—is a side effect well-known to cancer patients who take powerful drugs. The control group had taken, in essence, nothing at all, yet they experienced a marked physiological alteration."[16]

Bates wrote of the powers of suggestion and belief in the fitting of prescription lenses. People would claim to benefit from spectacles that had been prescribed improperly by others:

> In fact, many patients have told me that they had been relieved of various discomforts by glasses, which I found to be simply plane glass. One of these patients was an optician who had fitted the glasses himself and was under no illusions whatever about them; yet he assured me that when he didn't wear them he got headaches.
>
> Some patients are so responsive to mental suggestion that you can relieve their discomfort, or improve their sight, with almost

any glasses you like to put on them. I have seen people with hypermetropia wearing myopic glasses with a great deal of comfort, and people with no astigmatism getting much satisfaction from glasses designed for the correction of this defect.[17]

In a case reported in the medical literature, an optician had made a mistake in a prescription for prism lenses, used to compensate for eyes that turn inward or outward. The prescription ended up being the opposite of what it should have been. The person wearing the glasses never complained about them being a problem, so the error went unnoticed for quite some time. The researcher, according to Bates, explained the person's satisfaction with the incorrect glasses "by 'the slight effect of weak prisms and the great power of imagination'; and doubtless the benefit derived from the glasses was real, resulting from the patient's great faith in the specialist."[18]

As Meir Schneider notes, "Our eyes—and thus our visual abilities—are linked inextricably with our bodies, our minds and our emotions."[19] It's all a consequence of the strain syndrome, the mind/body adapting to the stresses thrown our way. Borrowing from a couple of common sayings, we could perhaps state, "Strain is in the eye of the beholder" and "You are what you think."

COLORFUL EMOTIONS

An ancient collection of Taoist stories and monologues contains the following passage: "Joy, anger, sadness, happiness, worry, lament, vacillation, fearfulness, volatility, indulgence, licentiousness, pretentiousness—they are like music issuing from hollows, or moisture producing mildew. Day and night they interchange before us, yet no one knows where they sprout."[20]

In our current digital age, we may have e-mail, e-commerce, e-business, and e-solutions, but *emotions* have been with us forever. Emotions, whether positive or negative, surface from the depths and ignite us to act in a certain way. When overcome with sadness, we say we are *moved* to tears. If the circumstances are happy, we might *jump* for joy. The moving aspect is, in fact, the derivation of the word *emotion,* Latin from *ex* (out of) + *movere* (to move). Our instinctive fight-or-flight response in dangerous situations is the very act of *moving out of* fear. We have to quickly decide, "Do I go after the beast (real or imaginary), or do I run away?"

Some psychologists suggest we are never without emotions; we supposedly fluctuate from one emotional state to another.[21] The emotional shifts apparently go on continually but are usually so subtle that we never consciously pay heed to them. It's only when we encounter circumstances that evoke stronger emotions that we suddenly become aware of the changes churning within our bodies. That's why we also call emotions *feelings,* because we literally feel them, from our very inner core to our outer skin, and from head to toe.

Through poetry, song lyrics, and day-to-day conversation, our language is replete with colorful symbolism expressing an array of emotions. Examples of common sayings include "feeling blue," "seeing red," "tickled pink," "mellow yellow," "green with envy," "good as gold," and "under a black cloud." During a fit of profanity someone is said to use "colorful language." If they're rattling off the words in quick succession, they're swearing a "blue streak." Under the heat of the moment, a person may suddenly drop a false persona and show their "true colors."

Artists have long been in touch with their emotions through the palette, but the use of colors dramatically changed during the Expressionist era in the late nineteenth to early twentieth century. It was an artistic movement that rose in opposition to the prevailing academic art standards of the day. The goal of the Expressionists was to display their inner feelings and emotions instead of depicting nature or reality as accurately as possible. One of the distinguishing factors was the use of wild and violent colors to convey the dynamic intensity of their innermost emotions. Vincent van Gogh was famous for his expressionistic style, particularly his self-portrait showing his missing ear. Interestingly, it has been speculated that van Gogh may have suffered from Ménière's disease, the severe inner-ear disorder discussed in the last chapter that causes such scrambling of the senses and resultant emotional turmoil.

Abstract art further pushed the envelope of emotional expression. Russian painter Wassily Kandinsky, considered one of the pioneers of this style, was also an accomplished musician. He said, "[I] applied streaks and blobs of colors onto the canvas with a palette knife and I made them sing with all the intensity I could." A harmonic link between colors and music—the integration of sight and sound—was an age-old idea that previously intrigued scientists like Newton. To further emphasize the connection between music, colors, and emotions, Kandinsky declared, "Generally speaking, colour is a power which directly influences the soul. Colour is the keyboard, the eyes are the hammers, the soul is the piano with many strings. The artist is the hand which plays, touching one key or another, to cause vibrations in the soul."[22]

In chapter 1, I touched on the serious impact of post-traumatic stress disorder (PTSD). An artist who was a Vietnam War veteran suffered severe depression coping with PTSD. During this period, his paintings were monochromatic, full of despair, terror, and gloom. After being treated with color light therapy, his paintings changed dramatically by incorporating many more colors. Dr. Robert Dubin, the clinician, noted, "His work now is lighter; it's brighter; it's more beautiful; it's more hopeful; and it's much more open."[23]

The very act of painting itself can be emotionally therapeutic. One of behavioral optometrist Roberto Kaplan's patients turned to painting as part of his vision therapy to help resolve repressed anger. "I became passionate about letting the paintbrush move effortlessly over the canvas," he said. "The strokes were the path for the anger to flow. I found the force of the inner volcano and it left me through my hands. I looked at the vibrant red and orange colors in front of me and felt relief."[24]

Johann Wolfgang von Goethe, the famous poet, dramatist, novelist, and scientist, conducted prolific experiments on the nature of light and color as documented in his 1810 publication, *Theory of Colors*. Goethe stressed the importance of both inner and outer light for vision: "The eye is formed by the light and for the light so that the inner light may emerge to meet the outer light."[25] His meshing of subjective and objective mirrored Plato's wisdom many centuries earlier. Physicist Arthur Zajonc observes, "According to Plato, the fire of the eye causes a gentle light to issue from it. This interior light coalesces with the daylight, like to like, forming thereby a single homogeneous body of light. That body, a marriage of inner light and outer, forges a link between the objects of the world and the soul."[26]

The classic teachings of color and color perception have been dominated by mechanistic theories and Newton's influence. Light could supposedly be reduced to simple component parts, quantifiable by means of different wavelengths. It was a tidy explanation that conveniently left out the dynamic interaction of the observer. There was nothing qualitative about it—simply objective physical phenomena. Quantum physicists are finding that Goethe was right. The observer and the observed mesh.

The conventional theory of color vision was seriously challenged in the 1950s, purely by accident. Edwin Land, inventor of the Polaroid camera, encountered a unique experimental situation that couldn't be explained by the existing concept of color perception. While projecting lights with different-colored filters on specific images, Land and his assistant could see a full spectrum of colors that hypothetically they shouldn't have been able to see. The traditional theory stated that they needed three filtered lights shining on the images to obtain the full hue of colors. They had only two colored filters. How did the eyes "fill in" the rest of the image to obtain the missing colors? Is it perhaps the projected light from the mind's eye of the observer meshing with the light rays of the outer image?

Over the rainbow lies your pot of golden sight, but you must follow the arc inward. Lao Tzu stated, "Using the outer light, return to insight."[27] Search your rich inner kaleidoscope of colorful feelings to help find your purity of vision.

HABITUAL SEEING

Fear, as we've stated already, is the most obvious emotion that gives us intense feelings, but there are other emotions, such as shock, surprise, anger, disgust, or contempt, that trigger certain physiological reactions. For example, with a strong emotion, the heartbeat immediately skyrockets, as does the rate of breathing. The digestive system grinds to a halt, and a sense of "butterflies" takes over. The mouth gets dry, the muscles shake, body temperature rises, and the senses become heightened.

Feelings at a less-extreme level maintain a strong influence on our muscles. Muscular contraction occurs in response to emotional stimuli; the muscles tense to get ready for action. Does a repeated stimulus create the so-called muscle memory that's responsible for stubborn habits and addictions? Consider smokers who try to quit. They'll unconsciously reach for a pack of cigarettes in their pocket that's not even there. Is it the nicotine itself that's most addictive, or is it more the feel of the various movements? Even though smoking is a vile, disgusting, and deadly habit, the various muscular actions involved—lighting a cigarette, holding it a certain way in the hand, caressing it with the lips, and inhaling and exhaling just so—is considered very pleasurable, perhaps sensual, to those so addicted. In fact, many smokers claim it's a form of relief from the effects of emotional stress. Similarly, joggers run even though injured to supposedly get the "endorphin high." But is the muscular movement just as addictive as the body's natural chemical substance?

The link between emotions and muscles is so powerful that the pleasure of indulging in unhealthy habits or activities outweighs the logic of knowing the potential or actual harm inflicted. As psychologist Paul Ekman states, "Emotions can override . . . the more powerful fundamental motives that drive our lives: hunger, sex, and the will to survive."[28] The limbic system seems to rule the roost over the R-system and neocortex.

Psychologist Albert Bernstein coined the alliterative phrase "Triple F response: fight, flight, or fright" to add a third dimension to the fear reaction. The "fright" response, he suggests, is different from the other two in that it involves no movement. This state is "stimulation overload" because it results in "blanking out and becoming immobilized, being unable to act, or restricting your actions," much like a deer frozen in the headlights of an oncoming vehicle.[29] For vision, this immobilization is what Bates referred to as staring, which was discussed in chapter 3.

It seems that test anxiety is an example of an addictive eye-muscle response that produces staring. Bates knew of many cases where vision would fluctuate with a change in emotional context. For example, a seamstress had no trouble threading a fine black thread through the eye of a needle, but she couldn't read small black print at the same distance. Similarly, a child could look out the window and easily make out all sorts of fine details in the distance, yet had trouble reading an eye chart only twenty feet away. In such cases, once the test anxiety was removed, the eye muscles "remembered" to see in a more dynamic and natural manner and acuity improved.

Ellen Langer undertook a study that showed how a slight change of context can influence visual acuity. The study involved subjects immersing themselves in the role of Air Force pilots. They all received a short physical exam, including an eye test, and then dressed in uniform. They were told to "be" pilots and actually took the controls of a flight simulator. While "flying" the simulator, the subjects had to look out the cockpit window to occasionally read markings on the wings. Unknown to the subjects, the markings were letters of different sizes from an eye chart. The result of this rudimentary experiment showed that for almost half the subjects, their vision improved! The conclusion: "Our perceptions and interpretations [via our senses] influence the way our bodies respond. *When the 'mind' is in a context, the 'body' is necessarily also in that context.*"[30]

The context in this sample study was one of assuming another personality. "All the world's a stage," according to Shakespeare. By taking the stage as pilots, who are known for their good vision, visual acuity improved for many subjects. The findings are not surprising in light of studies done on persons who have a multiple-personality disorder. People who suffer from this condition can have markedly different visual acuities from one personality to another. The same person may be tested as having 20/20 sight in one personality state, yet require prescription glasses in another state. The physical organs of sight are the same, but the context of character traits hugely influences the actual perception.

A wealth of information has been gathered correlating personality traits to specific visual conditions. The topic is beyond the scope of this book, but generally speaking, introverts are typically nearsighted, whereas extroverts tend to be farsighted. I'm oversimplifying here, but the dominant personality style is an individual's response to the environment, either suppressing or expressing a range of emotions. Your habitual emotional demeanor ultimately manifests itself in the eye muscles. Prescribing lenses may restore clarity artificially, but the lenses act as a negative reinforcement loop. The personality style habitually stays contracted.

Aesop's fable about a man, a boy, and a donkey teaches us that you can't please everyone. A corollary moral to me is that everybody sees things from a different emotional perspective. No two eyewitness accounts ever match detail for detail. In fact, law enforcement is relying less and less on eyewitness testimony as its trustworthiness has become increasingly suspect. Many people have been wrongfully convicted after they were picked out of a police lineup. The witnesses firmly believed the person they chose was the culprit.

Arthur Zajonc notes how context, experience, and insight shape the manner in which we see objects. The astute and passionate eye of a geologist looking at a rock outcropping sees something far beyond what Zajonc perceives. "I make a few distinctions, he a hundred, and each one tells a story to him of which I know nothing: glaciation, a lake bed, or volcanic lava flow; he finds the fossil under my foot. I feel not only illiterate but blind."[31] They both look at exactly the same object, yet the perception for each is completely different.

Michael Polanyi, philosopher of science and social science, describes how a similar "blindness" occurs during the initial stages of learning. For example, when a young medical student studying the diagnosis of pulmonary diseases first looks at a chest X-ray, he might only see "the shadows of the heart and ribs, with a few spidery blotches between them." The student is at first blind to the numerous features the experts seem to clearly see and discuss with zest and meaning. By observing more case studies and listening to his mentors day after day, the student gradually begins to see pathological signs and scars that weren't "there" to him earlier. "He still sees only a fraction of what the experts can see, but the pictures are definitely making sense now."[32] The proverbial light bulb clicks on inside the skull, and understanding clicks with it. A new habit has taken hold.

Regaining clear eyesight involves changing old patterns of sense perception. Even an anatomically perfect eyeball does not necessarily see perfectly. The medical literature has many cases where surgeons successfully corrected physical defects in congenitally blind* eyes only to discover the patients still couldn't see what the sighted take for granted. Although external light shone freely through their eyes and fully bathed their retinas, vision didn't fully click with them. They continued to rely on habitual modes of sense perception that were most comfortable to them: touch, hearing, and smell. The feeling of blindness was so deeply ingrained on a holistic scale that much of the blindness persisted with their "good" eyes. The act of seeing turned out to be a highly formidable process, not an automatic outcome expected by the doctors.† An eye surgeon lamented, "Education is the most important factor. . . . To give

---

*The term *congenitally blind* here does not refer to complete and utter blackness. In fact, such total blindness is rarely the situation for those categorized as blind. The patients generally had severe cataracts (opacity of the lenses) in their eyes, much like the childhood condition of Meir Schneider discussed in chapter 5. Had their retinas been dysfunctional for light reception, surgery would not have helped; restoration of their sight would have been impossible. The patients were functionally blind beforehand, meaning they could sense some light, and perhaps shadows or colors, but such perception was of little use. For all intents and purposes, they were as disabled as someone living in total blackness.

†In a more recent case study, it was interesting to note that the muscular movements in the patient's postoperative eyes were dysfunctional: "Searching eye movements were minimal, and when they did move over a large amplitude, they did so in larger than normal saccadic jerks which were plainly visible."[34] The act of seeing is far more than simply a matter of unobstructed light converging on the retinas.

back sight to a congenitally blind person is more the work of an educator than of a surgeon."[33]

EYE LANGUAGE

If actions speak louder than words, emotional *re*actions speak volumes. The face and eyes convey a universal form of nonverbal communication. Psychology professor and researcher Paul Ekman has been studying the relationship between facial expressions and emotions for many years. His research has confirmed that facial expressions triggered by common emotions are not culturally programmed. Even congenitally blind people make the same emotional facial expressions as those born with good sight. What *is* culturally learned is being stoic or attempting to hide the feelings—for example, putting on a brave face or a poker face. The permutations and combinations of the contraction of many different muscles in the face and head result in over ten thousand possible facial expressions.[35] (I wonder if comedic actor Jim Carrey can do all ten thousand.)

One of the most surprising results of Ekman's research was the inverse relationship of muscle contraction to emotions. Intentionally making a certain facial expression to mimic a particular emotion induces the very feelings of that emotion, whether it is sadness, anger, or joy. Science, then, has confirmed what Selye's grandmother told him when he was six years old and crying: "Anytime you feel that low, just try to smile with your face, and you'll see . . . soon your whole being will be smiling."[36]

When a person smiles, we sometimes remark how the eyes light up. The link between the eyes and facial expressions is, indeed, very apparent to an observer, especially for some of the common emotions that are considered negative—anger, fear, disgust, sadness, and contempt. You may not be able to read a book by its cover, but you can sure read a person's facial expression. Very few have the acting ability to hide instinctive and spontaneous muscular reactions. Here is a summary of some of the changes around the eyes for three of the most common negative emotions:[37]

Emotion	Eye Responses
Sadness	Inner corners of eyebrows pull together and up in the middle.
	Eyes look downward and upper eyelids droop.
	Eyes tear.
Anger	Eyebrows pull down and together, with inner corners toward the nose.
	Eyes open wide so that upper eyelids push against lowered eyebrows.
	Eyes have hard glare appearance.
Fear	Eyebrows pull together and raise as high as they can go.
	Upper eyelids raise as high as they can go.
	Lower eyelids tense slightly.

Eyebrow movements also occur when we are doing work involving intense effort. Eckman further notes that the expression "is produced by what [Charles] Darwin called the muscle of difficulty. He noticed, as I have, that any type of difficulty, mental or physical, causes this muscle to contract, lowering and drawing the eyebrows together. Perplexity, confusion, concentration, determination—all may be shown by this action. It also occurs when someone is in bright light, as the brows are lowered to act as a sunshade."[38]

The lowering and drawing together of the eyebrows also happens when someone is staring or straining to see. Squinting is another form of mental effort that Bates saw all the time. He could confidently predict that such an expression usually meant a lowering of the person's refractive state. Bates's 1920 book includes photographs of primitive and aboriginal people taken at the World's Fair in St. Louis. While looking at the camera with bewilderment and wonder, most were squinting and straining. Their perplexed classic eyebrow expressions led Bates to conclude they were most likely temporarily myopic at that point, even though their vision was tested as normal before the photo sessions.

Recall in chapter 3 how Bates had found that the refractive state would fluctuate under all sorts of emotional and physical discomforts, stresses that result in a strain on the visual system. Furthermore, he observed that when a person wasn't straining, the "muscles of the face and of the whole body are also at rest, and when the condition is habitual there are no wrinkles or dark circles around the eyes." But in cases of eyestrain, "the eye quickly tires, and its appearance, with that of the face, is expressive of effort or strain."[39]

Even in the absence of strong emotional reactions, the eyes themselves convey a great deal of nonverbal communication. In 1890, William James noticed that internal thought processes and eye movements are related. "When I try to remember or reflect, the [eye] movements . . . seem to come from the periphery inwards and feel like a sort of withdrawal from the outer world . . . [and] are due to an actual rolling outwards and upwards of the eyeballs."[40] Contemporary research in a field known as Neurolinguistic Programming (NLP) has expanded on that observation and, indeed, discovered that eye movements are anything but random. The various eye movements made while tapping our memory or imagination provide strong clues to inner thought processing. NLP contends the following relationships exist for right-handed people (left-handed people's responses are the mirror image):[41]

Eye Movements	Designation	Inner Processing
Up and left	Visual Remembered (VR)	Seeing familiar images
Up and right	Visual Constructed (VC)	Seeing creative images
Lateral left	Auditory Remembered (AR)	Hearing familiar sounds
Lateral right	Auditory Constructed (AC)	Hearing creative sounds
Down and left	Auditory Digital (AD)	Hearing your inner dialogue
Down and right	Kinesthetic (K)	Feeling imagined emotions, movement or touch

Recall in chapter 3 we discussed the rapid eye movement (REM) that occurs during sleep. REM activity may somehow be related to these same NLP designations. Recent findings reinforce the connectivity of the senses, particularly the strong relationship between sight and sound. As the writer Joseph Chilton Pearce explains it, "When we dream our eyes move. We used to think this was to follow the movement of the dream images but every movement of our eye muscles shifts the auditory fields of our brain. Shifting the auditory fields shifts our visual imagery. Spatial location and movement of images are part of the sight-sound dynamic within us. Our auditory function is directly involved in the construction of our three-dimensional world-space, the three dimensional objects filling that space, and movement of those objects in the resulting space."[42]

Our eyes are meant for far more than seeing and focusing on external objects. The vast extent to which the eyes and nearby facial muscles communicate and partake in movements day and night in response to emotions, memory, and visualization is astonishing.

MENTAL AND EMOTIONAL BALANCE

I've often wondered how many people with strong prescription lenses have to struggle with various anxiety disorders because of the relentless and continual emotional strain. That's because I've personally coped for years with phobias, particularly fear of heights and social-anxiety disorder. These conditions seemed to develop in my midteens, right around the time my progressive myopia peaked to near my strongest prescription. I also have photophobia, oversensitivity to strong light. It turns out there is a relationship after all.

Psychiatrist Harold Levinson has treated thousands of cases of learning disabilities and phobias and discovered a common physical correlation. Over *90 percent* of his patients who were dyslexic or phobic had a malfunction of the inner-ear system.[43] The vast majority of people with learning disabilities or phobias don't have some brain disturbance or disease entity; they simply have a hidden balance disorder.

A couple of decades before Levinson's work, an ear, nose, and throat physician in France made a strikingly similar discovery about the role of the ear in learning. Through his research on sound frequencies, Dr. Alfred Tomatis concluded that a listening problem is the root cause of such varied problems as attention deficit disorder (ADD), attention deficit hyperactivity disorder (ADHD), learning delays, autism, dyslexia, and sensory integration and motor skill difficulties. As Pearce notes, Tomatis found that the inner-ear system is a "principal congregating point for all our senses. Every neural process passes through or relates to this inner-ear complex. . . . Eye, head, and neck mobility have traditionally been associated with the optic nerve, but Tomatis found these functional structures 'under the control of the acoustic nerve . . . a major mechanism of reception and integration of perception.'"[44]

These findings are compelling evidence of somatic compliance: mind and matter go hand in hand. It confirms what Rudolf Steiner stated in 1923. Steiner, whose scholarly psychological and spiritual research led to a holistic, human-centered approach in the medical field (Anthroposophical Medicine), suggested that mental disorders are linked to physiological disorders. "But one will find over and again," he wrote, "that especially in so-called mental illness—which actually has been, as such, incorrectly named—physical processes of illness are present in a hidden way somewhere. Before one wants to meddle . . . with mental illness, one ought actually, with the proper diagnosis, to determine which physical organ is involved in the illness."[45]

Recall the array of potential symptoms of inner-ear dysfunction mentioned in the previous chapter. It's not surprising that many children and adults can have learning disabilities and high anxiety if they have to live with such jumbled sensory input and mixed-up coordination output. It raises the question, how many people wearing glasses have an undetected inner-ear disorder, no matter how slight?

Bates in his day recognized cases of students with learning difficulties, citing a case of one teacher who "had a class of children who did not fit into the other grades. Many of them were backward in their studies. Some were persistent truants." With the aid of simple eye-relaxation methods, the students were able to improve their eyesight and their studies. "At the end of six months all but two had been cured, and these had improved very much, while the worst incorrigible and the worst truant had become good students."[46]

The connection between stuttering and poor vision was also recognized back then. In 1927, a teacher of speech improvement observed firsthand, "Poor speech and poor sight often go together. . . . Those who stammer are invariably nervous, and the palming and swaying . . . calm the nerves and help the children to speak more quietly and slowly and therefore without stammering."[47] She had children practice Bates eye-relaxation techniques to treat their blurred vision and stammering at the same time. Peter Grunwald, the NVI instructor mentioned in the previous chapter, also stuttered from an early age. His speech difficulties improved in conjunction with his NVI program.[48]

INTEGRATING THE SENSES

Developmental and behavioral optometrists know that the eyes are not just for sight. They have confirmed that visual difficulties are connected to mental development and emotional behavior, with such problems as dyslexia, slow reading and poor comprehension, ADHD, and juvenile delinquency. The importance of integrating the senses with whole-body movements is a hallmark of this specialized field of optometry. Neurodevelopmental optometrist Merrill Bowan refers to these integration techniques as "mental gymnastics."

The training, which targets children with behavioral learning or reading difficulties, involves the use of a minitrampoline or rebounder. The goal is to develop "easy, automatic sequenced motor movements which are then combined with cognitive activities. . . . Marching, clapping, choral speaking, singing, dancing, workout videos . . . all have benefits."[49] The cognitive activities typically incorporate bouncing on the trampoline with rhythmic arm and hand movements and visual interaction with special wall charts. Or the child could be instructed to call out answers to rapid-fire mental tasks, like mathematics or spelling. Adults have also benefited from this type of training. Optometrist and NVI specialist Jacob Liberman calls it "effortless learning" and gave his first-hand positive experience in his book *Take Off Your Glasses and See.*

Based on Levinson's findings about inner-ear disorders and dyslexia, current treatment programs are being developed (reinventing the wheel, actually) that involve, lo and behold, movement. A program "has been taken up by 10,000 people at Dyslexia, Dyspraxia and Attention Treatment (DDAT) Centres in the UK, US and Australia. . . . Exercises are designed to 'train' the cerebellum to respond normally to information from the vestibular system." The exercises "might involve throwing beanbags and performing manual tasks while standing on one leg."[50] The psychology researchers conducting these studies found a significant improvement in reading, writing, and verbal fluency, as well as in reading comprehension.

Mary Bolles is a therapist who has had specialized training in NVI, sensory integration, whole-brain accelerated learning, and auditory integration training. She treats learning-disabled children and adults with the simultaneous use of light, sound, and motion.[51] A patient receives visual and auditory stimulation while lying on a comfortable cushioned surface that gradually moves (a motion table). The visual stimulus is in the form of colored-light therapy, and the auditory stimulus involves specific frequencies (based on the work of Tomatis) via stereo headphones. The motion table slowly rises and descends in a circular pattern to stimulate the vestibular system. The post-treatment results show remarkable improvements. The peripheral visual field expands noticeably, hearing anomalies improve, and learning difficulties abate. Some children no longer require prescription glasses afterward. It's hard to say which of the three stimuli has the most impact. Regardless, it's truly an integrated approach.

Craniosacral therapy (CST), briefly mentioned in chapter 6, has proven to be valuable in treating hyperactive and dyslexic children. With hyperactivity, osteopath John Upledger found the culprit was usually a jammed occipital bone, where the base of the back of the skull joins the neck. Once the CST treatment had released the "stuck" area, the craniosacral system returned to normal functioning and the hyperactive behavior subsided. The success rate for such cases at the time was nearly 100 percent.[52] For dyslexics, Upledger found the problem area to be near the ear in the temporal bone. Scores of children improved their reading and academic skills after CST treatments. The success rate was an impressive 70 percent.[53]

British osteopathic physicians have also found a relationship between the inner ear, the TMJ, and dyslexic symptoms. A combination of cranial osteopathy and vestibular treatment was thus developed. Cranial osteopathy, which was actually the basis for the development of CST treatment, involves manipulating the TMJ and skull plates near the ear region to make these areas more flexible. The vestibular treatment involves twirling, tossing, and tumbling the children in numerous gentle ways to get the inner ear free and fluid.[54]

HEART OF THE MATTER

The physicist and philosopher Blaise Pascal was famous for stating, "The heart has its reasons of which reason knows nothing." A segment of the scientific community is now recognizing that the heart is, indeed, smart. Joseph Chilton Pearce comments on this intelligence of the heart: "Transmitters, which play such a critical role in neural behavior, have now been found in the heart and are connected in some way with the brain. . . . We now know that the heart . . . controls and governs brain action through hormonal, transmitter, and possibly finer quantum-energies of communication."[55] Famous heart surgeon Christiaan Barnard apparently once suggested that medicine had to give up the idea of an artificial heart because the organ is more than a pumping station.

The ancient art of massage has long recognized that bodywork is more that just physical therapy on aching muscles and joints. Releasing physical tension has a way of uprooting old emotional blockages, especially when working near the chest area. Meir Schneider explains:

It is interesting that the muscles of the chest (and also of the arms) may often be extremely tender to the touch even when they do not hurt or ache otherwise. . . . [A] very important feature of this region is the extent to which emotions appear to be "stored" there. . . . Many bodyworkers have observed that massage of the chest, and often of the arms, can produce a great uprush of emotional expression and release, and that a person with very tense and tender chest muscles will often prove to have been carrying a burden of unexpressed emotion which the massage can do much to relieve. It is no coincidence that the heart has been named as the seat of emotion.[56]

Wilhelm Reich, a classically trained psychoanalyst, applied the Freudian technique called *free association* in his clinical practice with limited success. This method of encouraging the patient to speak freely about psychological problems has long been caricatured: the patient reclines on the couch and says whatever comes into his or her mind, while a monocled therapist takes notes, occasionally asking probing questions in a thick Viennese accent. By observing his patients' demeanor and whole-body posture, Reich detected a common "armoring" that was indicative of suppressed emotions. He chose to break ranks with his Freudian roots, reconnecting the artificial mind/body division. Incorporating bodywork during the therapy sessions helped patients unleash old emotional blockages, usually with high energy and intensity. His work developed into Reichian therapy and offshoots such as Bioenergetics. Janet Goodrich and other NVI therapists successfully employed these emotional-release techniques in conjunction with Bates's eye-relaxation methods.

A therapist simply acts as an intermediary, helping individuals connect with their hearts. The physical touch can be very gentle and subtle, guiding a patient into a meditative/hypnotic-type state that initiates the self-healing process. As part of his massage-therapy practice, Upledger developed adjunct modalities, called SomatoEmotional Release and Inner Physician, which he found to be very powerful. A patient intuitively assumes a body position that seems to gradually release stored-up emotions from the tissues. "There may be crying, shaking, sweating, laughing, pain . . . almost anything you can imagine. . . . It gives them recall of experiences, traumas, accidents and the like that they have been holding beneath the surface of their awareness for years."[57] Following Upledger's guidance, a woman managed to reverse her worsening symptoms of glaucoma with such an inner-centered process. The puzzled eye doctor thought there must have been a mistake in the original tests, for when he remeasured the fluid pressure in her eyeballs, the value was almost normal.[58]

The goal of these various therapies is to help a person get to the heart of the matter. According to ancient Chinese medicine, all of us, regardless of sex, have a mixture of mental and emotional qualities inherited from our parents that are evident in each side of the body. The left side holds the feminine (yin) side of our character—intuition, imagination, creativity, feeling, spontaneity, artistic ability, and so forth—while the right side is the masculine (yang) side—logical, analytical, deductive, linear, planning, scientific, and so on. Is it any coincidence that the word *matter* is derived from the Latin word *mater,* meaning "mother," and that the heart is on the left side of the chest? The "heart of the matter" is literally being attuned to the nurturing, emotional side.

The right/left attributes also manifest themselves through the eyes. Roberto Kaplan makes use of this important concept in a couple of unique ways: iris analysis reading and eye patching. Suppressed emotion leads to muscle tension. The likelihood of a person suppressing emotion can be analyzed from the emotional structure of the iris, the colored part of the eye. Not only do emotions get stuck in the muscles, they literally show up in the irises, the colored portion of the eyes. Kaplan incorporates integrated iris reading analysis as part of his Integrated Vision Therapy. When, as a professor of optometry, he was first introduced to iris reading analysis, he was highly skeptical. Once he began mapping personality patterns in patients' irises, he was pleasantly surprised to find the method to be about 80 percent accurate. Patients were typically taken aback that he could so accurately predict that behavioral traits that arose were highly correlated to unresolved emotional wounding. Using the information gleaned from the irises, he helps patients get to the root of their visual problems. Typically the patients recognize and release old blocked fears and angers, stripping away layers of a "survival" persona—essentially the Reichian armoring previously described—to find their "true essence" or "soul presence."[59] The other right/left concept involves wearing an eye patch over the dominant eye. If someone is overly rational and analytical (as most myopic people are), Kaplan encourages patching the right eye for extended periods at home each day (while doing safe activities that do not depend on having binocular vision). The person automatically becomes more aware of the feeling side of vision. Various emotions and memories can come to the surface, facilitating the goal of more integrated seeing.

Active meditation (meditation combined with visualization and affirmations) such as the Silva Method is another means to assist people in ridding themselves of negative emotional patterns that block healing energy. Martin Brofman has firsthand experience. In 1975 he was diagnosed with terminal cancer and given only one to two months to live. The emotional jolt and feeling of initial hopelessness was nothing like he'd ever experienced. He eventually met a Zen master who said, "Cancer begins in your mind, and that's where you can go to get rid of it."[60] That's just what he did. Not only did he cure himself of his cancer, the amazing and unexpected side benefit was restoring vision. For twenty years he had worn prescription eyeglasses for myopia and astigmatism, yet once he was cancer free he was also lens free. His soul journey completely transformed his life as well. He traded his old Wall Street career and lifestyle for one of dedication and service, creating the Brofman Foundation for the Advancement of Healing.

Emotional healing through an NVI program generally requires some assistance. As Kaplan suggests, "It is very important to have a trained person assist you. Counselors, psychologists, psychiatrists, psychotherapists, vision therapists, Bates teachers, vision educators, and rebirthers are good choices. Ask a friend to be a support person as well." There are many other holistic modalities too numerous to mention that help unlock deep-seated emotions that may be a barrier to continued improvement. Find a method that feels right for you, because they all achieve the same goal in the end. I've personally encountered emotional healing via massage therapy and from a holistic practitioner who specializes in a powerful technique called Theta Healing. The spontaneous and intense emotional releases were as shocking as my first clear flash of vision. Daily meditation and affirmations have become newly acquired habits. A further cathartic process has been writing this book, moving away from my logical and mathematical bent to a more creative and intuitive side.

ANOTHER REALM

I was about to play a golf game on an unfamiliar course. One of my playing partners was a friend with whom I hadn't had a golf round in about a dozen years. The other two in the foursome were strangers. I was last to hit my drive from the first tee box as the others watched and waited. I teed up my ball and took my swing with the driver. I could immediately feel from the feedback in the grip that I had "skied" the shot, in what is known as a pop-up drive (this type of mis-hit results in a shot going farther vertically than it does horizontally toward the hole). I was embarrassed that I'd skied it so badly. My playing partners were not impressed and waited impatiently for the ball to land. I sheepishly asked, "Has it come down yet?" My friend sneered and responded, "No, it hasn't." At that point they all promptly decided to desert me; they left the tee box and headed in a direction away from the first hole.

Abandoned on the tee box, I waited some more and finally heard the sound of a ball hitting the ground. I followed the sound over toward the right side of the fairway. Once there, I could see literally hundreds of balls scattered all over the place, much like at a driving range. But I knew this wasn't the driving range. As I approached the balls, I looked at one, then another, and yet another. None of the balls was mine. I kept this up for a brief period and soon realized in frustration that I probably wasn't going to find my ball. It was like looking for a needle in a haystack.

I then decided to walk in the opposite direction toward the left side of the fairway and into the rough. While walking through the longer grass, I came across a ball. I knew this wasn't where I had heard my drive land, but I thought, "Maybe this is my ball." I picked up the ball and looked at it closely. It wasn't just a standard white ball with the usual dimple pattern. It was emblazoned with a very intricate pattern. Each dimple was a different shade of gray with a fine, black-lined, hexagonal border. I'd never seen a ball like it before. Although it had an unusual pattern, the ball did have a regular logo on it. The logo was the familiar "Hogan" signature seen on that manufacturer's line of golf equipment.

The next thing I knew, a man was walking toward me. He was a middle-aged black man carrying a set of golf clubs. I asked him, "Is this your ball I found?" He came over, took a look at the ball, and said, "Yes, that'll be mine." He thanked me, took his ball, and walked away without even playing his next shot.

Did this really happen? Not during my waking hours, but during my sleeping hours. I saw it and experienced it as a weird dream one morning before rising. As I was eating breakfast, I recalled the dream and suddenly realized what it meant. It wasn't about golf at all, but about vision improvement. Here's how I interpreted the imagery:

Teeing up and hitting a driver represented my goal of improved vision by natural means.

The "skied" tee shot represented the goal as "up in the clouds" and unrealistic by the orthodoxy.

The long time the ball was in the air symbolized that NVI takes time and that much patience is needed.

The playing partners who left me represented the public and orthodox vision practitioners who ridicule and reject NVI, so I felt very much alone in my quest.

Looking for the ball on the right side of the fairway represented practicing two Bates fundamentals: shifting and concentric focus.

The rough on the left symbolized the perseverance required for NVI.

Looking at the intricacies of the unique ball also represented shifting and concentric focus to see the fine details.

The right and left images of each side of the fairway represented the
teamwork of both eyes for integrated vision.

Famous pro golfer Ben Hogan was nicknamed "The Hawk" for the
fierce look in his eyes when competing in his prime; the logo
represented the keen, hawklike eyesight that would eventually
be mine.

The black man, about my age, represented freedom from glasses.

This was the most cryptic vision dream I'd had to that point. Many
of my other vision dreams required no interpretation; they would tend
to have a recurring theme and setting related to vision improvement. For
example, I would be in a dimly lit room noticing the blurry surroundings, when I would say to myself, "This is crazy, I can see just fine!"
The dream scene would immediately become clear, and I could see the
finest details. Vision dreams are a common occurrence with NVI, demonstrating that the healing process goes beyond the physical realm and
the waking state.

Esoteric teaching might attribute this healing to the continuous
activity of the soul. As Rudolph Steiner noted, "The soul lives in a higher
world, just as the physical body lives among the things and beings of
the physical world, where it is affected by them and works upon them.
But the soul's life continues during sleep. Indeed, the soul is particularly
active then . . . the soul draws the inspirations and impulses by means of
which it works unendingly on the physical body."[61] Although the inner
continuously impacts the outer, for most people, it is an unconscious
process while awake, a unity of spirit, soul, and body in harmonious
concert with the mysterious and imperceptible Tao.

Look, it cannot be seen—it is beyond form.
Listen, it cannot be heard—it is beyond sound.
Grasp, it cannot be held—it is intangible.
These three are indefinable;
Therefore they are joined in one.[62]

PART THREE

HARMONY

Knowing harmony is called constancy,
knowing constancy is called clarity.

LAO TZU

8

VIRTUE

The highest Virtue seems empty;
Great purity seems sullied.

For the countenance of great virtue,
only the Way is to be followed.

LAO TZU[1]

For argument's sake, let's say I've never had a daydream and have no idea what a daydream is. Other people tell me that they see and hear things vividly in their heads at various times throughout the day. It's much like reality, but it's not *out there* where you can actually grasp it. You've got to be kidding me! Inside your head? You even have songs playing over and over that you heard earlier in the day on the radio? I don't believe it for a minute! There's no scientific evidence to support such an outlandish and preposterous suggestion. There may be instruments that display waves and blips on a monitor to signify brain activity. But daydreams? I suppose you see fairies dancing on pinheads, too!

NVI is commonly charged with being unscientific. (Actually anything is unscientific if scientists refuse to study it.) That's enough to raise skeptical concerns and deter many people from taking it seriously. Yet there are so many common experiences we share that could be deemed equally unscientific. We take it for granted that everyone else has them, so we conclude they must be factual and true. We let our senses judge what is reality and what isn't. But for some reason, we're led to believe we're unqualified to judge for ourselves how our most valuable sense of eyesight fluctuates naturally and how clarity returns on its own if given a chance. You must taste it yourself, for the proof really is in the pudding.

In this day and age, science has attained the stature of a highly virtuous endeavor. It's considered the pinnacle in the quest for and discovery of truth, the very core of material progress. The standard of living enjoyed by industrialized nations attests to scientific achievements. Along with this wealth and prosperity resides public faith in the positive role of science. Yet as discussed in chapter 1, there is a seedy side to technological advances. By trusting the scientific system and experts, we've lost our senses, so to speak. Science was intended to be a tool to enhance our sense experience for a better understanding of the world around us, not a method for replacing (or restricting) our senses.

To counter the skeptics during his day, Bates's writings included social commentary about scientific dogma, mass-produced education, and rigid thinking in general. It revealed an intriguing aspect of the man beyond his medical training.

WHY

A young woman cut off a small slice of roast before placing it in the pot to cook. A friend who was visiting at the time asked her why she cut the slice beforehand. The woman replied that she was simply following a customary practice of her mother's, but she didn't really know why. The woman decided to phone her mother to ask the same question. The mother replied that she'd learned this preparation technique from her mother. Still curious, the woman next phoned her grandmother to find out if she knew. The grandmother indeed had the reason: "Because that's the only way it would fit in my pot."[2]

Bates seriously questioned why the eye-care profession continued to keep "cutting another slice" in the treatment of visual blur. But Bates wasn't just questioning tradition for the sake of curiosity, nor did he intentionally set out to be a troublemaker. Having found a better way in vision care, he felt a moral obligation and duty to speak out. Alexander Solzhenitsyn, the Soviet dissident who spent many years as a political prisoner during the iron rule of Stalin, wrote: "The simple step of a courageous individual is not to take part in the lie. One word of truth outweighs the world." Bates took the bold step of uncovering the *eye lie* and paid a terrible price, personally and professionally. He may not have been sent to a correction camp, but he was as good as exiled in his own land. Sadly, his principles and teachings continue to be mostly underground practices to this day.

Bates was of the view that most scientists appreciated the limits in their quest for discovery, knowing there always remained a great deal of uncertainty. Sir Isaac Newton, considered by many to be one of the forefathers of science, may have agreed. When he developed his law of gravity, he really only explained *how* gravity worked in mathematical terms, not *why*. Newton's critics at the time were quick to point out that he never really "discovered" gravity. Since it couldn't be detected by the senses, it was essentially an occult property. In a private letter to a friend, Newton admitted that gravity may have innate and mystical properties, for he felt its cause could be an "immaterial agent."[3]

Newton entertained this view because he was not an emotionally detached materialist as science textbooks would like to portray. Much like the spin-doctors in this day and age, science writers tidied up Newton for the public. When Newton's descendants auctioned off his private manuscripts in 1936, famous economist John Maynard Keynes was surprised when he read the contents. The "science" in which Newton immersed himself was much broader than what we understand the field to encompass nowadays, for he was obsessed by the science of the occult. His writings showed that he was grounded in Hermeticism, an ancient wisdom tradition that believed consciousness and matter are one. He studied the sacred geometry of the pyramids and undertook alchemy experiments. Alchemy, the intriguing discipline that psychologist Carl Jung revisited from a current-day perspective, was a major part of Newton's life, as he maintained an extensive alchemical library.

Newton was a deeply spiritual man who apparently believed he was a chosen prophet of his generation. He read divine meaning into two potentially fatal circumstances in his life. The first occurred when he was not expected to live after his premature birth in a parish that had a high infant mortality rate. The date he was born was Christmas. Years later as a young man, he again beat the odds when he escaped contracting the deadly plague. In one of his alchemical textbooks he inscribed a phrase that is translated as "Jehovah the holy one."[4] As science and technology historian Lewis Mumford points out, "It is not, perhaps, an accident that most of the great spirits in science, from Kepler and Newton to Faraday and Einstein, kept alive in their thought the presence of God—not as a mode of explaining events, but as a reminder of why they are ultimately as unexplainable today to an honest enquirer as they were to Job."[5]

I consider Bates to be a "great spirit" in vision science whose peer recognition is long overdue. He was well aware that life was largely shrouded in mystery and that science has its limits in determining what can ultimately be known. With all the technological advancements and research that has occurred since Bates's day, the vision industry seems no further ahead than where it was in 1921:

> The causes of disease are obscure and variable, and we do not know it all. It does not seem to me that a doctor is justified in telling a patient that he is incurable just because he has never seen such a case cured, or has forgotten, because it was contrary to rule, any case that he has seen. This may cause the patient to accept as inevitable a condition which might have been cured, and may even prevent Nature, because of the depressing effects of discouragement, from doing what the doctor has failed to do. Still less is it justifiable for the medical profession to assume, as it now seems to do, that we have learned all there is to be known about blindness.[6]

Vision science continues to be obsessed with studying the mechanics of the eye—"how" it works, "how" vision becomes blurry, and "how" to treat poor vision artificially. Bates stepped away from that obsession to ask, "Why?" This led him onto a completely different path, one that nature had provided in the first place—self-healing. He knew full well where the credit lay in the vision-healing process. When someone asked him what his method was, he was hard pressed for an answer: "Many people have asked me what I call my treatment. The question was a very embarrassing one because I really have no name to give it unless I can say that my methods are the methods employed by the normal eye. When a person has normal sight the eye is at rest, and when the eye is at rest, strange to say, it is always moving to avoid the stare."[7] In other words, he humbly admitted he was simply helping people attain clear vision by retraining them in the natural use of their eyes.

KNOWLEDGE

Taoist sentiments toward knowledge at first glance appear quite strange, the antithesis of Bacon's famous statement, "Knowledge is power":

> *In the pursuit of learning, every day something is
> acquired.
> In the pursuit of Tao, every day something is
> dropped.*[8]

The contemporary application of Bacon's maxim is to use knowledge for a competitive edge in careers, sales, and business, especially in our era of computers and the information explosion. In contrast to this view of knowledge, consider the following anecdote from cultural historian Morris Berman:

> When my maternal grandfather turned five, he was sent . . . to the
> . . . Jewish elementary school. . . . It was the custom . . . that each
> boy was given a slate upon entry. . . . It was his personal possession,
> on which he would learn to read and write. And on that first day,
> the teacher did something quite remarkable: he took the slate, and
> smeared the first two letters of the Hebrew alphabet . . . in honey.

As my grandfather ate the letters off the slate, he learned a message that was to remain with him all his life: *knowledge is sweet.*[9] [Emphasis added.]

Quite a contrast, isn't it? Sweet instead of powerful. Formal, acquired knowledge is indeed important; but it's also to be appreciated and cherished, not simply used for manipulative self-gain or controlling purposes.

Whether you think knowledge is powerful or sweet, the acquisition of knowledge is only a narrow segment on the broad spectrum of all forms of understanding. What about instinct, intuition, imagination, creativity, foresight, dreams, and the like? Are these not forms of intelligence that give us greater meaning? Taoism certainly contends this to be the case:

> *Always passionless, thereby observe the subtle;*
> *ever intent, thereby observe the apparent.*[10]

"Subtle" in the first line refers to "formless intuition," knowledge that is implicit and unconscious. "Apparent" in the second line refers to "discursive intellect," knowledge that is explicit and conscious.[11] To give you everyday examples of these two concepts, consider how preschool-age children acquire knowledge.

Toddlers are not given formal lessons on how to speak. They aren't instructed on the proper use of the lips, tongue, throat, or palate to produce various sounds. They aren't given the meaning of words, vocabulary, or rules of sentence structure. Instead, they intuitively start to pick up a few words and gradually develop a vocabulary. Not only that, they manage to string together words at random to formulate their own unique statements or questions. This is truly implicit learning. The explicit, intellectual part comes later when children enter school and are formally taught to read and write. This second stage of learning is a very rational, logical process with clearly defined rules, according to linguist W. Nelson Francis: "The rules of grammar, particularly those of the native language, are, as it were, invented by the child as he learns the language; they are largely unconscious, self-invented, and self-imposed. Only if he should happen to study formal grammar much later in life will the speaker encounter explicit formulations of these rules, and even then he may not recognize them. It seems rather paradoxical that many people find the study of grammar difficult, when all it is is an attempt to formulate what they themselves invented when they were children!"[12]

Taoism is paradoxical in many ways, but the philosophy has a perspective on learning and knowledge that's broader than this explicit view. Taoism further suggests the mysterious "subtle" is the more useful form of knowledge on the broad spectrum. To Taoists, it's infinite, a deep well that never runs dry. Einstein put it similarly when he stated, "Imagination is more important than knowledge. Knowledge is limited. Imagination encircles the world." By comparison, the Western approach is that rational or scientific knowledge is the only type of knowledge worthy of serious consideration.

PURE SCIENCE?

What guiding principles establish your beliefs and help you make important decisions? Do you have to see it to believe it? Or do you depend on expert opinions or seek out persons with credentials? Maybe you have complete faith in the Bible and the word of God. Perhaps you just intuitively "know" that a certain direction is your calling in life.

Hunter Lewis, author of *A Question of Values*, suggests we all have a number of value systems that guide us in shaping beliefs and making choices, but when push comes to shove, we're typically motivated by a dominant system. He postulates that we use the following core value systems: authority, deductive logic, sense experience, emotion, and intuition. Interestingly, he adds science as a sixth category, even though it's a combination of the others. (The scientific method uses intuition to develop a hypothesis, logic to develop the experimental test procedures, sense experience to observe the findings and collect data, and logic to draw conclusions.)

He included science in his framework because it is a dominant value system in our industrialized society for many people. We are trained to be skeptical of any claim unless science proves it to be "true." If the scientific experts give a claim their blessing, skeptics can lower their guard and rest assured the claim is credible. But what exactly is this "science" that is so high and mighty? According to Lewis, there are three gradations of scientific knowledge, from the purest to the highly questionable:[13]

Exact science. Meets all the following stringent conditions: the facts must be clearly and objectively stated (with no hidden bias); the key research variables must be independent (not all mixed together with other variables); experimental procedures must be measurable and repeatable (anyone following the same steps should get exactly the same results).

Inexact science, quasi–science, or "science." Generally relies on a combination of experience, intuition, and logic, but falls short of meeting all the conditions of exact science.

Pseudoscience. Pretends to be scientific but is not even completely factual or logical. Hence a confused or even fraudulent attempt to wrap oneself in the prestige of exact science.

The term *exact* is somewhat presumptuous and misleading, because it implies purity and total objectivity. It invokes an image of men and women in lily-white, starched laboratory coats surrounded by test tubes, twisting dials on shiny, metallic equipment to make brilliant discoveries, all the while emotionally detached and free of bias. To suggest that exact or pure science exists is like saying the *Titanic* was unsinkable. There is no more total objectivity in science than there is in journalism. People can certainly strive for such lofty goals. But face it; there is always human bias, whether it's conscious or subconscious, that affects the outcome or the spin taken. It may not seem initially apparent even under close scrutiny, but you just can't escape the fact that humans come with a myriad of fantasies, follies, and frustrations.

Furthermore, the criterion noted for *exact* in this definition is based on a dated assumption. This premise introduces an immediate bias by stating that variables can be completely isolated and independent of one another, suggesting the whole is nothing but an assemblage of parts that have no interrelationships. Science, having begun with this vantage point, has ironically found quite the opposite to be the case.

Newer branches of physics and mathematics have completely undermined the original scientific premise. Christopher Bache, professor of religious studies and researcher of deep consciousness, notes the profound insight these disciplines provide is "the discovery that parts cannot be meaningfully isolated from the systems in which they exist. In the subatomic world of quantum mechanics and the macro-world modeled by non-linear mathematics, *all individual, particulate existence shows itself to be inseparable from its corresponding fields.* Individual pieces of life cannot be realistically isolated from their surrounding matrix. Not only is it impossible to do so except as a rough approximation, but at a deeper level it is misguided to attempt it."[14]

These radical new views from the scientific community are a consequence of the nature of the scientific process itself. Karl Popper, a renowned professor of logic and scientific method at the London School of Economics, contended that science was essentially a work in progress. Discovered "truths" are tenuous and fleeting. Geneticist David Suzuki, in a similar vein, writes, "The very nature of science is that most of our current ideas are wrong, irrelevant or unimportant. Science progresses by demonstrating that our hypotheses and conjecture need to be overhauled, thrown out or modified."[15] Alfred North Whitehead, the English mathematician, logician, and philosopher, put it succinctly: "Knowledge does not keep any better than fish."

Unfortunately, the tendency to attribute eternal truth to scientific findings seems to create a built-in bias to ignore anomalies or exceptions. If certain phenomena occur but are calculated to be statistically insignificant, then they're brushed aside and forgotten. Bates, in contrast, treasured exceptions to rules; he had the ability to find a diamond in the rough. Holistic physician Dr. Larry Dossey says, "Nature seems to be shouting, 'Here lies the treasure! Dig here!' But we [doctors] have . . .

allowed narrowness . . . to replace awe and wonder."[16] It's those very gems that are necessary for a radical shift in thinking and to explore fresh new possibilities.

Harold Levinson was another doctor who had the ability to break free from scientific conformity, to find a hidden treasure in the puzzle of dyslexia and phobias. Even after practicing as a clinical psychiatrist for several years, he considered himself scientifically naïve, thinking the experts were always right. But eventually other developments and ideas crystallized with his work, starkly contrasting with existing theories. He found much of the scientific literature to be erroneous, some even "fictitious." Much of it "had little to do with science—at least little with what I knew and felt science to be." He concluded "scientists did not always have the grasp of their science that they should have had . . . that I was taught they had."[17]

Much of this type of scientific debate can go on without widespread public knowledge. But sometimes stories come to the forefront. You've probably read a medical news story outlining a type of diet that is good for you only to read another story later stating how bad the diet is for your health. If you use science as your dominant value system in guiding your beliefs and actions, where do you side? Which expert is "right?"

Vision science is particularly fraught with fragmentation that befuddles the public. It has a long history of dissension and uncertainty that raises the question of just how pure the science has been to date. There are competing professional bodies with their own unique educational training, research goals, and treatment methods, all vying for your business. Politics and turf wars come into play.

Traditionally the two main camps are ophthalmologists (medical doctors or MDs) and optometrists (doctors of optometry or ODs). The science of ophthalmology is the medical model, concerned with eye disease and offering treatment with lenses, drugs, or surgery. The science of optometry evolved from the physics model and is concerned with the mathematics of optics and refraction. "Corrective" lenses were offered to offset refractive errors within the eye.

The two distinctly scientific viewpoints have been feuding much like the Hatfields and McCoys for the past century. The dissension reached a head in 1965 when the American Medical Association (AMA), representing the ophthalmologists, tried to officially boycott the business of optometrists. The optometrists countered with an antitrust lawsuit, and the AMA was ultimately forced to dissolve its resolutions. The rivalry over scope of practice continues to this day. Ophthalmologists and optometrists are now clashing over who has the right to perform laser eye surgery.

A specialized group of ODs, called behavioral/developmental optometrists, has branched out to create its own niche. This third group is the most holistic, and many of these professionals are not only familiar with Bates's work and NVI but several have had success in applying his principles. Unfortunately, they constitute a small minority within the marketplace and are spread thinly among the population. As a result, the public is largely unaware of their work because very few people have access to their services.

EDUCATIONAL CLONES

John Amos Comenius was considered one of the founders of the modern school system during the seventeenth century. He envisioned that his proposed schooling would provide a perfect outcome: "It will be as pleasant to see education carried out on my plan as to look at an automatic machine, and the process will be as free from failure as these mechanical contrivances when skillfully made."[18]

Charles Dickens didn't see the outcome of such utilitarian, mass-manufactured education in quite the same light. Dickens's searing 1854 satire, *Hard Times,* included the character of Mr. M'Choakumchild, a young graduate schoolmaster who, along with "some one hundred and forty other schoolmasters, had been lately turned at the same time, in the same factory, on the same principles, like so many pianoforte legs. He had been put through an immense variety of paces, and had answered volumes of head-breaking questions. . . . If he had only learnt a little less, how infinitely better he might have taught much more!"

The consequences of this utopian attempt to stamp young minds in repeated mass-production fashion certainly didn't go unnoticed by Bates either:

> You may force a few facts into a child's mind by various kinds of compulsion, but you cannot make it learn anything. The facts remain, if they remain at all, as dead lumber in the brain. They contribute nothing to the vital processes of thought; and because they were not acquired naturally and not assimilated, they destroy the natural impulse of the mind toward the acquisition of knowledge, and by the time the child leaves school or college, as the case may be, it not only knows nothing but is, in the majority of cases, no longer capable of learning.[19]

This educational compulsion to force-feed the same curriculum requires compliant students. They must have faith that what they are learning is factual. Acclaimed British mathematician and biologist Jacob Bronowski, who developed a BBC television series on the history of science, commented on faith—or lack thereof—in education. He noted a tradition at a very old and respected German university, a bastion of leading-edge scientific research. "The University is a Mecca to which students come with something less than perfect faith. It is important that students bring a certain ragamuffin, barefoot irreverence to their studies; they are not here to worship what is known, but to question it."[20]

Such irreverence is more of a rare commodity in most modern universities geared toward cranking out degrees for the work world. The mass-manufactured mindset of these institutions relies heavily on the faithfulness of their students. Most students are content in the role of sponges, soaking up the information without question. What background would impressionable young people have to be suspicious or critical of technical and specialized course content? And besides, what choice do they have but to trust the curriculum completely? Why would they even think of risking repercussions from professors, possibly putting their future careers in jeopardy? The cloning process of like-minded students thus continues year after year based on a conditional response. Ellen Langer explains:

> We are taught about *theories, models, hypotheses,* and not just "facts." Theories and the like are implicitly conditional and explicitly statements of uncertainty. . . . If a theoretical model is presented absolutely, it will be thought absolute and the student may thereafter treat it rigidly. . . . Scientific investigations yield only probability statements and not absolute facts. And yet, these probabilistic data and information that are true only under certain circumstances are presented in textbooks as though they were certain. . . . If something is presented as an accepted truth, alternative ways of thinking do not even come up for consideration. . . . By teaching absolutes we pass our culture from one generation to the next. It brings stability. But . . . the cost may be high.[21]

In chapter 3, we touched on Bates's preference for empirical facts over theories. Contemporary physicists also refer to empirical science as *exploratory experimentation* and suggest that this style of research has been ignored for too long "by historians and philosophers of science . . . [but] has nevertheless played a crucial role in the history of physics."[22] Michael Faraday, considered one of the greatest scientists of the past two centuries, favored empirical experimentation to theoretical experimentation. So great was his work that Einstein celebrated him as one of two scientists who had the most profound role in changing the face of physics since the era of Newton. Physicist Arthur Zajonc explains Faraday's experimental style:

> From his earliest researches in science, Faraday possessed a love for truths gotten through direct experience, and consequently he held an abiding distrust of speculative theories. . . . Ever aware of the danger of such speculation in his own research, Faraday penned the following entry in his diary for December 19, 1833. . . . "I must

keep my researches really *Experimental* and not let them deserve any where the character of *hypothetical imaginations.*" The key word here is "hypothetical." Time and again new ideas and imaginations must be grounded in honest experimental fact, otherwise fantasy takes the place of cautious creative thinking.[23]

Theories, models, and hypotheses become accepted as dogma among researchers long before they reach the classroom. Beth Savan, a Canadian environmental scientist, studied the political realities in science to show how the system is biased in favor of existing theories. Before a scientific study can be published, it must pass a peer review. This is the stage when other scientists study the report and its conclusions and try to pick it apart. If it passes the review, the findings are published. Originally a safeguard built into the system to ensure integrity, peer review has gradually come to thwart much innovation. Savan contends peer reviewers and journal editors are usually like-minded types who favor established views, whether intentionally or not. Scientific journals, she says, "can become doctrinaire, deliberately eschewing challenges to accepted theories." Journals support certain lines of thinking, so the peer-review process usually creates an "Old Boy network of successful scientists with power to determine research priorities, promote favoured theories or hypotheses, and make or break academic careers."[24]

Ian Stevenson, early in his career as a medical researcher in biochemistry, would have encountered this very resistance had he attempted to publish a research report in another country. He and his colleague obtained unexpected experimental data that effectively destroyed the dogma of a great German chemist, Otto Warburg. Their report was published locally in the United States. "I thought little of that," he wrote, "and was astonished one day when a German biochemist who learned of our results told me that it would have been impossible to publish them in Germany. He meant that the awe in which Warburg was held would have led to editorial rejection of our report."[25]

Also keep in mind that science is, first and foremost, a business; dollars and prestige drive research and development (R&D). The most lucrative direction for R&D scientists is typically the path of least resistance. Such a choice involves a leap of faith. Savan observes, "In every aspect of their work, scientists rely heavily on the techniques, methodology, knowledge, and theories developed by their colleagues. If they hope to advance their field, they must build on previous work—and must assume that their predecessors did the experiments they claimed to have done, and reported their results accurately."[26]

As with any profit-making venture, the age-old human temptation to fast-track fortune and fame can sometimes lure a scientist off the ethical path and send him or her skidding toward academic transgressions. Such unscrupulous activity—typically perpetuated by individuals who had previously been highly respected in their fields—occasionally comes to light in the media.* How much skullduggery goes undetected is unknown, especially if experimental results are "tweaked" ever so slightly to massage statistical data for the desired payoff. Notes David Suzuki, "If scientists are willing to employ exaggeration, deceit or dishonesty merely for greater fame, promotion or acceptance to medical school, we can only speculate on what people will do under pressure from venture capitalists and vast sums of money."[27]

Vision science—presumably conducted mainly on the up-and-up—relies on anachronistic knowledge that is riddled with erroneous theories and contradictions. Each generation of neophytes willingly accepts the doctrine without question. Concerned about the continual acceptance of errors in eye education, Bates in 1920 wrote the following: "It is incomprehensible that men calling themselves scientific, and having had at least a scientific training, can be so foolish. One might excuse a layman for such irrational conduct, but how men of scientific repute who are supposed to write authoritative textbooks can go on year after year copying each other's mistakes and ignoring all facts which are in conflict

---

*Early in 2006, the media reported two cases of high-profile scientific fraud within a month of each other. In the East, a South Korean veterinarian fabricated cloning research, while in the West, a Canadian doctor world-renowned for his expertise in nutrition, allergies, and immunology was found to have concocted reports published in prestigious journals dating back to the 1980s.

with them is a thing which reasonable people can hardly be expected to understand."[28]

More and more studies in the same vein may generate a great deal of R&D interest and investment, but such a direction doesn't necessarily translate into groundbreaking work. Morris Berman notes, "It is an immense irony that the 'information explosion' of the modern era actually represents a *contraction* of our knowledge of the world."[29] It's much like what Lao Tzu said: "The farther you go, the less you know." The exponential growth in scientific studies and papers that quickly gather dust and totally fade into oblivion is truly quite dramatic, as noted by Lewis Mumford:

> Beginning with a single scientific journal in 1665 . . . there were a hundred at the beginning of the nineteenth century, a thousand by the middle, and ten thousand by 1900. We are already on the way to achieve 100,000 journals in another century. . . . The exponents of mass production of knowledge have created a hundred journals devoted only to abstracts of papers; and now a further abstract of all these abstracts has been proposed. At the terminal stage of this particular solution, all that will be left of the original scientific or scholarly paper will be a little vague noise, at most a title and a date, to indicate that someone has done something somewhere—no one knows what and Heaven knows why.[30]

Bates commented about endless studies that seemed to lead nowhere: "Voluminous statistics were collected . . . and are still being collected. The subject [of blurred vision] has produced libraries of literature. But very little light is to be gained from the perusal of this material, and for the most part it leaves the reader with an impression of hopeless confusion."[31] Optometrist Joseph Kennebeck lost his faith in optometric journals, saying he "was never interested or impressed by [scientific journal] articles. . . . I have already read most of them, and I see no reason for reading them again and again in articles written by others who had little or nothing else to say."[32]

Educational cloning continues to be a thriving business in the new millennium. Dickens's M'Choakumchild would be beaming with pride, for his creed that students "never wonder" lives on.

BLIND RULING THE BLIND

Our free society gives us the false sense of security that we are somehow safe from dictatorships or authoritarianism. That's because we tend to equate this sort of rule with government politics and sinister delusions of grandeur; such connotations are further reinforced in the media. For example, on the CBS television show *60 Minutes* not long ago, Andy Rooney commented about the danger of dictatorships shortly after the capture of former Iraqi leader Saddam Hussein:

> We congratulate ourselves all the time on our democracy here in America and for not having had a dictator. I don't know whether we've been lucky or smart. It could happen.
>
> The people who follow an evil leader don't have to be evil themselves. They can be dumb, uninformed, disinterested in the world, or just too absorbed with their personal problems to care about their government. It's been amazing, really, that this great democracy of ours has lasted so long.
>
> A dictator doesn't usually just come in and take over. He moves in little by little.[33]

Sorry to break the news, but it has happened. No, not a ruthless government dictator, but an authoritarian medical system. The authorities have taken over little by little throughout the centuries, and the system succeeds largely because of the very public attitudes Rooney described. Ivan Illich, author of *Limits to Medicine*, called this sort of authoritarian dominance of healthcare a "radical monopoly." It's an economic juggernaut which demands that people relinquish their capacity for self-care, self-coping, and self-healing, enslaving them to an iatrogenic social and cultural order:

Medicine is a moral enterprise and therefore inevitably gives content to good and evil. In every society, medicine, like law and religion, defines what is normal, proper, or desirable. . . . The physician decides what is a symptom and who is sick. He is a moral entrepreneur, charged with inquisitorial powers to discover certain wrongs to be righted.

Society has become a clinic, and all citizens have become patients . . . constantly being watched and regulated to fall "within" normal limits.

. . . The physician acts primarily as an actuary, and his diagnosis can defame the patient, and sometimes his children, for life. By attaching irreversible degradation to a person's identity, it brands him forever with a permanent stigma.[34]

This sort of inquisitorial zeal—diagnosing illness instead of health, ever eager to impose the latest vogue procedure—was exposed in New York as early as 1934.[35] Doctors examined a group of 390 children and selected almost half for a tonsillectomy. The rejected children were then examined a second time by a different group of doctors who were unaware of the results of the first examination. Roughly half of those children were chosen for the tonsillectomy. The process was repeated once more, and again almost half were selected for the operation. At that stage, only sixty-five children remained who were rejected for the procedure. Had the supply of doctors available for the examinations not run out, all the children likely would have eventually been selected.

The tonsillectomy has since fallen out of fashion and is now considered an unnecessary and invasive procedure. Unfortunately, the eye-care industry remains stuck in this bygone era; the zest for such diagnostic bias and treatment continues unabated, as evidenced by the alarming vision epidemic discussed in chapter 2. The radical monopoly quantitatively defines "normal" vision and insists that everyone must fit within that norm. Not only are we reduced to a number in this process, the final number imposed on everyone must be the same!

If you try to break free from the system, it comes with a price. Eye doctors and patients who embark on more natural alternatives come under attack. That's the other way authoritarian rule prospers—by carefully crafted propaganda. The most outspoken critics of Bates and NVI are typically self-appointed, fronting as "consumer advocates." It's easy to spot them by their usual propaganda ploys:[36]

> *Name calling.* This is the most blatant tactic, where labels of "quackery," "unscientific," "charlatan," and "cult," to list a few, are applied, and Bates's personal and professional character is attacked. Similarly, those who follow NVI are labeled "gullible" or "neurotic."
>
> *Glittering generalities.* This is the opposite of name calling, with the liberal use of "virtue" words about which people have deepset ideas; terms such as *progress, research, technology, science, doctor,* and *medicine* are used to promote a positive, reassuring spin.
>
> *Card stacking.* This deceptive device uses overemphasis, underemphasis, or distortion to evade the real issues.

Imre Lakatos, a distinguished mathematical and scientific philosopher, spoke of the predictable response to challenges to orthodox theories: "Scientists have thick skins. They do not abandon a theory because facts contradict it. They normally either invent some rescue hypothesis to explain what they then call a mere anomaly and if they cannot explain the anomaly, they ignore it, and direct their attention to other problems."[37]

Many obviously go a step further than simply ignoring contrary new facts; they circle the wagons and direct their attention to challengers in a hostile manner. Nutritionist Gary Null and physician Debora Rasio write, "All 50 states have enacted strict proscriptions at the state medical board level against using so-called unscientific medicine, meaning anything that is not, according to the orthodox consensus, common-use medicine. Hundreds of physicians have been prosecuted and punished for not confining their treatments to the accepted paradigm, some to the point of having their licenses revoked, being imprisoned, or suffering bankruptcy. And it has been of only secondary importance whether or not their patients have claimed to benefit from their treatments."[38]

The specter of such draconian measures has haunted NVI practitioners for decades. Most prominent was the 1940s court case of Margaret Corbett, who ultimately was found not guilty of practicing medicine or optometry. Although she was spared a conviction, the net result was to drive NVI and the Bates Method largely underground. Janet Goodrich and colleagues—practitioners who went public in the 1970s—found themselves taunted by authorities who threatened to take similar types of legal action. In fact, Goodrich eventually moved to Australia to resume her practice in an environment free of continual intimidation.

These sorts of authoritarian responses are incredibly far removed from legitimate scholarly debate. As Bates himself said of aggressive defensiveness and posturing, "Such dogmatism is both unwise and unscientific . . . [and] throttles research."[39] Skepticism is a hallmark of the field of scientific endeavor. But skepticism doesn't imply guarding current theories as immutable and treating anomalies and exceptions with contempt. The skepticism must apply first and foremost to currently accepted scientific theories. As Lakatos emphatically stated, "Blind commitment to a theory is not an intellectual virtue: it is an intellectual crime." Why such a strongly emotional statement from a scientist? He knew what society ultimately accepts as scientific truth "has grave ethical and political implications."[40]

The consequences in medical science are indeed grave. The establishment is profiting from orthodox treatment while at the same time putting the public at undue risk. Null and Rasio undertook an eight-year review of over ten thousand medical studies taken directly from such well-recognized sources as the *Journal of the American Medical Association,* the *New England Journal of Medicine,* and *The Lancet.* The review concluded that the "vast majority of medical procedures are done with the *belief* [emphasis added] that they are safe and effective, rather than with [scientific] proof that they are. Even after procedures and medications have been shown (a) not only not to work, but (b) to cause injury and death at a statistically significant level, they continue to gain in popularity and use."[41]

A similar unfounded belief in efficacy and safety prevails in orthodox vision care, even when the scientific evidence points to the currently accepted treatments being iatrogenic. The vision specialists know full well their products do not cure blurred eyesight, and they are literally turning a blind eye to the damaging outcomes. The deeply entrenched eye-care industry continues to grow and prosper, while the safer, natural, holistic alternative is mocked on the sidelines.

Our two eyes work together to merge visual data in a unified image, with greater clarity, depth perception, and perspective, than monovision. Such a unified image desperately needs to develop between the opposing sides of vision-care providers.

CONCLUSION

Excess is confusion.
Therefore sages embrace unity
as a model for the world.

The Way for humans
is to act without contention.

LAO TZU[1]

COMMON SENSE AND PURPOSE

It's been said that if common sense were so common, a lot more people would have it. We do have it, but it largely goes unused when we defer to authority figures. The first step in gaining back some common sense is to realize that you are a consumer, and not a patient, of medical goods and services, and that eye doctors and their ancillary supply houses have something to sell you. Whether the goods and services are purchased by Medicare, a private insurance company, or out of your own pocket is immaterial. Are you getting value for the dollar?

We spoke in the previous chapter of the fragmentation within the eye-care industry. This type of splintering is prevalent in the medical sciences in general. For the sake of the consumer, there needs to be more common sense and common ground among the professional disciplines.

John Mew (who happens to be dyslexic) faced suppression in the field of orthodontics and dentistry for his new ideas concerning naturally guiding facial growth. He comments on the dilemma in the medical sciences: "In years gone by . . . issues could be debated in an open forum such as the British Royal Society, where a wide range of views would be expressed by separate scientific disciplines and obvious inconsistencies addressed. However, there is now no . . . body to oversee common sense in science."[2]

If that were a start, then hopefully such a governing body would represent the public by including holistic practitioners and laypersons. Such individuals, who are not part of the clique but possess a strong sense of altruism and ethics, may be best able to see the big picture. Commenting on the endless debates about technological risk assessment, Harold Lewis commendably admitted a similar view: "It is painful for a scientist to say this, but we do sometimes get so involved in arguing technical nuances that only a less well-informed person can make any decision at all."[3]

Morris Berman contends that conventional science as we know it has run its course, although he agrees that intellectual analysis is a very important human tool, despite its abuse. He claims we are at a stage in history where we need to develop a postmodern science that is more holistic—one that reunites twins that should never have been separated in the first place: *objectivity* and *subjectivity*. He sees the work of Gregory Bateson, the famous cultural anthropologist, social scientist, and cyberneticist, as representing such a holistic science, which places a strong emphasis on the social and natural environment. Berman explains: "As scientific civilization enters its period of decline in earnest, more and more people will search for a new paradigm, and will undoubtedly find it in various versions of holistic thinking. If we are lucky, by 2200 AD the old paradigm may well be a curiosity, a relic of a civilization that seems millennia away."[4]

Gregory Bateson was influenced by the broad thinking of his father, William Bateson, a well-known biologist who coined the now household word *genetics* in 1906.* The elder Bateson viewed the organism

---

*I find it a remarkable and fitting coincidence that the name William Bateson is strikingly similar to the name of the holistic eye doctor, William Bates, and that the two men were born within a year of each other.

as a whole and reasoned that when a local variation occurred, such a variation would affect the entire organism. His holistic views extended to learning as well, for he believed that true education was much more than merely a dull, utilitarian preparation for a numbing career. He also maintained that science was an artistic pursuit, an endeavor that was never meant to be emotionally cold and detached. Yet he noted it was easier for a scientist simply to solve problems than feel them as a poet or painter would.

The division between the two sides to health and healing is no longer as clear-cut as it once was. If we apply the adage "united we stand, divided we fall," then we're still very wobbly in gait. But there are many dedicated men and women employed in the orthodox medical industries who have much more progressive views than their counterparts of a generation or two ago. After all, they are consumers of curative medicine, too, and they want to do what's best for their health and the health of their loved ones. The holistic side to health is justly gaining momentum and support in mainstream thinking, as envisioned by Berman:

> There will be a strong shift in medical practice toward popular and *natural healing;* an avoidance of drugs and chemical manipulation; and a near merger with ecology and psychology, since it will be widely recognized that most disease is a response to a disturbed physical and emotional environment. Birth will not take place on the "assembly line" of the modern hospital, but at home. . . . The body will be seen as part of culture, not a dangerous libido to be kept in check. . . . This future culture will also see a revival of the extended family. . . . The elderly will be mixed in with the very young, rather than dumped in old-age homes . . . and their wisdom will be a continuing part of cultural life.[5] [Emphasis added.]

This shift to holism is taking place, albeit at a seemingly glacial pace because of the prevailing elitist politics—the defenders of orthodox vision science (Us) versus holistic practitioners and laypersons (Them). Actor and comedian Steve Martin took a jab at this sort of division in a parody about gaining membership in an elitist organization: "Joining Mensa instills in one a courtly benevolence toward nonmembers, who would pretend to know what you know, think what you think, and stultify what you perambulate. I worried about the arbitrary 132 cut-off point, until I met someone with an I.Q. of 131 and, honestly, he was a bit slow on the uptake."[6]

With over a couple centuries of vision science and very little to show but confusion, marketing of noncurative merchandise, and a growing epidemic of poor vision, exactly which side is "slow on the uptake"? Let's all get onstream with NVI, shall we?

> *The highest good is like water.*
> *Water gives life to the ten thousand things and does not*
>   *strive.*
> *It flows in places men reject and so is like the Tao.*[7]

NOTES

INTRODUCTION

1. Lao Tzu, *Tao Te Ching,* trans. Feng and English, chaps. 64 and 41.
2. Smith, *World's Religions,* 196–220.
3. Benjamin, *Better Sight,* 17.
4. Lao Tzu, *Tao Te Ching,* chap. 24.
5. Bowan, "Stress and the Eye."
6. Brumer, "Eyestrain."

CHAPTER 1: THE CHASE

1. Lao Tzu, *Tao Te Ching,* trans. Cleary, chap. 12.
2. Chen, *The Tao Te Ching: A New Translation with Commentary,* 204.
3. Ibid., 41.
4. Cleary, *Essential Tao,* 138.
5. Bates, *Cure of Imperfect Sight,* 4.
6. Nearing and Nearing, *Good Life,* 3, 13.
7. Ibid., 6.
8. Sahlins, "Original Affluent Society."
9. Ibid.
10. Selye, *Stress Without Distress,* 42.
11. Mumford, *Pentagon of Power,* 324.
12. Lao Tzu, trans. Feng and English, chap. 29.
13. Suzuki, quoted in Mills, *Turning Away,* 106.
14. Shelton, *Natural Hygiene,* 260.

15. Selye, *Stress of Life*, 50.

16. U.K. Department of Social Security, *Stress Related Illness*, part 1.

17. Selye, *Stress Without Distress*, 35.

18. Lightle, ed., "Cancer," 8.

19. U.K. Department of Social Security, *Stress Related Illness*, part 1.

20. National Mental Health Institute (NMHI), "The Numbers Count."

21. NMHI, "Depression Can Break Your Heart."

22. NMHI, "Reliving Trauma."

CHAPTER 2: LOSS

1. Lao Tzu, *Tao Te Ching*, trans. Feng and English, chap. 30; trans. Cleary, chap. 9.

2. Huxley, *Art of Seeing*, 20.

3. Bates, *Cure of Imperfect Sight*, 4–8.

4. Ibid., 8.

5. Ibid., 2.

6. Ibid., 99.

7. Kavner and Dusky, *Total Vision*, 40.

8. MacFarlane and Martin, *Glass*, 152.

9. Ibid.

10. MacFarlane and Martin, "Preliminary Drafts."

11. Huxley, 21.

12. Vision Council of America, "Sales, Purchase Intent."

13. National Academies' Institute of Medicine, "To Err Is Human," 26–27.

14. Nicolas S. Martin, "Promoting Accountability."

15. Eisenberg et al., "Trends in Alternative Medicine."

16. Bates, *Cure of Imperfect Sight*, 81–82.

17. Kennebeck, *Why Eyeglasses Are Harmful*, 86.

18. Huxley, 36–37.

19. Raphaelson, *Spectacle Hobby*.

20. Quoted in Raphaelson.

21. Druker, *Optical Journal*.

22. Kaplan, *Seeing Without Glasses*, xvi.

23. Brumer, "Eyestrain."

24. Canadian National Institute for the Blind, "Client Statistics 2002."

25. Selye, *Stress Without Distress*, 26.

26. Ibid., 22.

27. Quackenbush, *Relearning to See*, 32.

28. Centers for Disease Control and Prevention (CDC), "*Fusarium* Keratitis" and "Update."

29. Ibid.

30. Booth, "Eye Surgery Risks."

31. Feynman, *Space Shuttle Challenger Accident*.

32. Link, "Why We're Here."

33. Link, "Complications."

34. Rach2 [username], "Lonely and Frustrated."

35. Association of Vision Educators.

36. Bates Association for Vision Education.

CHAPTER 3: RHYTHM

1. Lao Tzu, *Tao Te Ching*, trans. Cleary, chap. 29; trans. Feng and English, chap. 55.

2. Chen, *Tao Te Ching*, 127–28.

3. Lao Tzu, trans. Feng and English, chap. 2.

4. Orlock, *Know Your Body Clock*, 7–8.

5. Zajonc, *Catching the Light*, 279.

6. Pulos and Richman, *Miracles and Other Realities*, 204.

7. Liberman, *Light*, 33.

8. Preidt, "Eye-Opening British Study."

9. Lao Tzu, trans. Feng and English, chap. 32.

10. Hirshberg and Barasch, *Remarkable Recovery*, 72.

11. Mumford, *Pentagon of Power*, 70, 394.

12. Bates, *Cure of Imperfect Sight*, 12–14.

13. Ibid., 21.

14. Ibid., 75–76.

15. Ibid., 75.

16. Ibid., 76.

17. Goodrich, *Natural Vision Improvement*, 5.

18. Bates, *Cure of Imperfect Sight*, 78.

19. Ibid., 77.

20. Liberman, *Light,* 84.

21. Gottlieb, "Neuropsychology of Myopia."

22. Kaplan, *Conscious Seeing,* 12.

23. Brown, "History of the Origin."

24. Bowan, "Toward a Unified Theory."

25. Liberman, *Take Off Your Glasses and See,* 89.

26. Quackenbush, *Relearning to See,* xxvi.

27. Beresford et al., *Improve Your Vision,* 47.

28. Bates, *Cure of Imperfect Sight,* 107–8.

29. Bates, "Vice of Concentration," 4.

30. Bates, *Cure of Imperfect Sight,* 107.

31. Ibid., 109.

32. Ibid., 98–99.

33. Bowan, "Stress and the Eye."

34. Kavner and Dusky, *Total Vision,* 24.

35. Bates, *Cure of Imperfect Sight,* 277.

36. Ibid., 257–8.

37. Bowan, "Stress and the Eye."

38. Bates, *Cure of Imperfect Sight,* 106, 276.

39. MacFarlane and Martin, *Glass,* 161.

40. Ibid., 161–63.

41. Peat, "Creativity and Education."

42. Bates, "Optical Swing," 9–10.

43. Bates, "Vice of Concentration," 7.

44. James, *Talks to Teachers.*

45. Gottlieb, "Neuropsychology of Myopia."

46. Huxley, *Art of Seeing,* 25–26.

47. Bates, *Cure of Imperfect Sight,* vii.

48. Bates, "Common Sense," 5.

49. Bates, *Cure of Imperfect Sight,* vii.

50. Huxley, *Art of Seeing,* 22–23.

51. Bowan, "Integrating Vision."

CHAPTER 4: SOFTNESS

1. Lao Tzu, *Tao Te Ching,* trans. Chen, chap. 76; trans. Feng and English, chap. 78.

2. Miller, *Triumphant Journey,* 21.

3. Keepin, "David Bohm."

4. Peat, "Blackfoot Physics."

5. Keepin, "David Bohm."

6. *Encyclopedia Britannica Online.* s.v. "Heracleitus." www.britannica.com (accessed January 4, 2004).

7. Selye, *Stress Without Distress,* 136.

8. Smith, *World's Religions,* 207.

9. Mitchell, *Tao Te Ching,* viii.

10. Huxley, *Art of Seeing,* 24–25.

11. Cole, *Pride and a Daily Marathon,* 62.

12. Smith, *World's Religions,* 209–10.

13. Bowan, "Integrating Vision."

14. Frost, "Two Tramps."

15. Selye, *Stress Without Distress,* 88.

16. Selye, *Stress of Life,* 422.

17. Bittman, "Deep Within."

18. Berenyi, "Healthy Rhythms."

19. Bittman, "Deep Within."

20. Bates, *Cure of Imperfect Sight,* 101.

21. Ibid.

22. Ibid.

23. Davies, *Trigger Point Therapy,* 30.

24. Selye, *Stress of Life,* 413.

25. MacDonald, *Alexander Technique,* 12–15.

26. Bates, *Cure of Imperfect Sight,* 113.

27. Quackenbush, *Relearning to See,* 3.

28. Huxley, *Art of Seeing,* 25.

CHAPTER 5: RETURN

1. Lao Tzu, *Tao Te Ching,* trans. Feng and English, chap. 40; trans. Chen, chap. 16; trans. Cleary, chap. 52.

2. Mihoces, "You've Got to See."

3. Ibid.

4. Bates, "Routine Treatment," 517.

5. Quackenbush, *Better Eyesight*, 517.

6. Bates, *Cure of Imperfect Sight*, 159–60.

7. Ibid., 160.

8. Kavner and Dusky, *Total Vision*, 9.

9. Lao Tzu, trans. Feng and English, chap. 29.

10. Bowan, "Integrating Vision."

11. Bates, *Cure of Imperfect Sight*, 161–62.

12. Ibid., 159.

13. Ibid., 166.

14. Colebrook, "Emergence."

15. Bates, *Cure of Imperfect Sight*, 114–15.

16. Ibid., 116–17.

17. Ibid., 115.

18. *MSN Encarta Online*. s.v. "Eye (anatomy)." http://encarta.msn.com/encyclopedia_761564189_1____3/Eye_(anatomy).html#s3 (accessed January 24, 2004).

19. Bates, "Shifting," 6.

20. Bates, "Routine Treatment," 5.

21. McCaffey, "Burning, Stinging, Gritty Eyes?"

22. Givens, "Eye Blink."

23. Lierman, "Individual Treatment," 16–18.

24. Bates, "Shifting," 6.

25. Peat, "Creativity and Education."

26. Kavner and Dusky, *Total Vision*, 76.

27. Bates, *Cure of Imperfect Sight*, 148–52.

28. Ibid., 101.

29. Ibid., 123.

30. Ibid., 170.

31. Ibid., 166.

32. Ibid., 118.

33. Ibid., 165.

34. Schneider and Larkin, *Handbook of Self-Healing*, 184.

35. Ibid., 186.

36. Orfield, "Seeing Space."

37. Huxley, *Art of Seeing*, 10.

38. Bates, *Cure of Imperfect Sight*, 88.

39. Ibid., 103–5.
40. Ibid., 218.
41. Kiesling, "Signs of Progress."
42. Kavner and Dusky, *Total Vision,* 43–44.

CHAPTER 6: BALANCE

1. Lao Tzu, *Tao Te Ching,* trans. Mitchell, chap. 77.
2. Calvert, "Mystery of the Senses."
3. Abrams, "Eyes in the Back of Your Mouth."
4. National Institute on Deafness and Other Communication Disorders, "Ménière's Disease."
5. Levinson, *Phobia Free,* 226.
6. Ibid., 98.
7. Ibid., 243.
8. Ibid., 287.
9. *WrongDiagnosis.com.* "Symptom: Blurred Vision."
10. Bates, "Tension," 4.
11. Cole, *Pride and a Daily Marathon,* 20–21.
12. Ibid.
13. Ibid., 129.
14. Ibid., 135.
15. Ibid., 130.
16. Levinson, 241.
17. Bates, *Cure of Imperfect Sight,* 83–88.
18. Bates, "Tension," 3.
19. Bates, "Lesson from the Greeks," 4.
20. Lierman, "Stories from the Clinic," 14.
21. MacDonald, *Alexander Technique,* 40.
22. Selye, *Stress of Life,* 414.
23. MacFarlane and Martin, Glass, 159.
24. Prudden, *Pain Erasure,* 69–70.
25. Beresford et al., *Improve Your Vision,* 32–33.
26. Davies, *Trigger Point Therapy Workbook,* 31.
27. Ibid., 30.
28. Ibid., 48.

29. Klemons, "Chest Pain and Headaches."

30. National Research Council, *Myopia*, 25.

31. Schneider and Larkin, *Handbook of Self-Healing*, 193.

32. Schneider, *Self-Healing*, 30.

33. Goodrich, *Natural Vision Improvement*, 37.

34. Gottlieb, "Neuropsychology of Myopia."

35. Bates, "Tension," 5.

36. MacDonald, *Alexander Technique*, 10, 16.

37. Grunwald, "Profile."

38. Orfield, "Seeing Space."

39. MacDonald, *Alexander Technique*, 37.

40. Cole, *Pride and a Daily Marathon*, 26.

41. Schneider and Larkin, *Handbook of Self-Healing*, 193.

42. Kiesling, "About the Webmaster."

43. Bates, *Cure of Imperfect Sight*, 122.

CHAPTER 7: WHOLENESS

1. Lao Tzu, *Tao Te Ching*, trans. Feng and English, chap. 39, chap. 10.

2. U.K. Department of Social Security, *Stress Related Illness*, part 2.

3. Leviton, *Seven Steps*, 58.

4. Twain, "Blind Tom."

5. Lao Tzu, trans. Mitchell, chap. 20.

6. Lewin, "Is Your Brain Really Necessary?"

7. Pearce, *Evolution's End*, 42–45.

8. Steiner, *Theosophy*, 29.

9. Ibid., 31.

10. Ibid., 32.

11. Langer, *Mindfulness*, 171.

12. Levinson, *Phobia Free*, 112.

13. Lao Tzu, chap. 11, personal interpolation of various translations.

14. Langer, *Mindfulness*, 192.

15. Cousins, *Anatomy of an Illness*, 69.

16. Hirshberg and Barasch, *Remarkable Recovery*, 73–74.

17. Bates, *Cure of Imperfect Sight*, 86.

18. Ibid., 87.

19. Schneider and Larkin, *Handbook of Self-Healing,* 186.

20. Cleary, *The Essential Tao,* 70.

21. Ekman, *Emotions Revealed,* 19.

22. Kandinsky, *Concerning the Spiritual in Art.*

23. Dubin, "Post Traumatic Stress Syndrome," 127.

24. Kaplan, *Conscious Seeing,* 194.

25. Zajonc, *Catching the Light,* 205.

26. Ibid., 21.

27. Lao Tzu, trans. Feng and English, chap. 52.

28. Ekman, *Emotions Revealed,* xvii.

29. Bernstein, *Dinosaur Brains,* 27, 34.

30. Langer, *Mindfulness,* 177.

31. Zajonc, *Catching the Light,* 204.

32. Berman, *Reenchantment of the World,* 138.

33. Zajonc, *Catching the Light,* 6.

34. Gregory and Wallace, *Recovery from Early Blindness.*

35. Ekman, *Emotions Revealed,* 14.

36. Selye, *Stress of Life,* 409.

37. Ekman, *Emotions Revealed,* 95, 134, 160.

38. Ibid., 138.

39. Bates, *Cure of Imperfect Sight,* 117.

40. James, *Principles of Psychology,* chap. 10.

41. Robbins, *Unlimited Power,* 128–33.

42. Pearce, *Evolution's End,* 70–71.

43. Levinson, *Phobia Free,* 17.

44. Pearce, *Evolution's End,* 71.

45. Steiner, *Polarities in Health.*

46. Bates, *Cure of Imperfect Sight,* 263–64.

47. Bates, "School Teacher's Report," 16.

48. Grunwald, "Profile."

49. Bowan, "Integrating Vision."

50. Young, "Controversial Dyslexia Treatment."

51. Bolles, "Learning Abilities' Dramatic Response," 297–318.

52. Upledger, *Your Inner Physician,* 25.

53. Ibid., 27.

54. Pearce, *Evolution's End,* 73.

55. Ibid., 103–4.

56. Schneider and Larkin, *Handbook of Self-Healing*, 23.

57. Upledger, *Your Inner Physician*, 79.

58. Ibid., 118–21.

59. Kaplan, *Conscious Seeing*, 65.

60. Brofman, *Improve Your Vision*, 12.

61. Steiner, *Higher Worlds*, 172–73.

62. Lao Tzu, trans. Feng and English, chap. 14.

CHAPTER 8: VIRTUE

1. Lao Tzu, *Tao Te Ching*, trans. Feng and English, chap. 41; trans. Cleary, chap. 21.

2. Langer, *Mindfulness*, 44.

3. Berman, *Reenchantment of the World*, 43.

4. Ibid., 120.

5. Mumford, *Pentagon of Power*, 121.

6. Bates, "Blindness," 9.

7. Bates, "Common Sense," 3.

8. Lao Tzu, trans. Feng and English, chap. 48.

9. Berman, *Reenchantment of the World*, 267.

10. Lao Tzu, trans. Cleary, chap. 1.

11. Cleary, *Essential Tao*, 132.

12. Francis, "English Language," 22a–23a.

13. Hunter Lewis, *Question of Values*, 110–11.

14. Bache, *Dark Night, Early Dawn*, 156.

15. Suzuki, "Erratic Journey."

16. Dossey, "Foreword," in Hirshberg and Barasch, *Remarkable Recovery*, xii.

17. Levinson, *Phobia Free*, 214–15.

18. Mumford, *Pentagon of Power*, 103.

19. Bates, *Cure of Imperfect Sight*, 106.

20. Bronowski, *Ascent of Man*, 360.

21. Langer, *Mindfulness*, 35, 127–28.

22. Ribe and Steinle, "Exploratory Experimentation."

23. Zajonc, *Catching the Light*, 134.

24. Savan, *Science Under Siege*, 119–20, 148.

25. Stevenson, "Journeys in Medicine."

26. Savan, *Science Under Siege*, 90.

27. Suzuki, "Erratic Journey."

28. Bates, "Prevention of Myopia," 8.

29. Berman, *Reenchantment of the World*, 268.

30. Mumford, *Pentagon of Power*, 174–75, 181.

31. Bates, *Cure of Imperfect Sight*, 251.

32. Kennebeck, *Why Eyeglasses Are Harmful*, viii.

33. Rooney, "Saddam's Capture."

34. Illich, *Limits to Medicine*, 45–46, 90, 166.

35. Ibid., 93.

36. Delwiche, "Propaganda."

37. Lakatos, "Science and Pseudoscience."

38. Null and Rasio, "Iatrogenic Illness."

39. Bates, "Blindness," 9.

40. Lakatos, "Science and Pseudoscience."

41. Null and Rasio, "Iatrogenic Illness."

CONCLUSION

1. Lao Tzu, *Tao Te Ching*, trans. Cleary, chaps. 22 and 81.

2. Mew, "Common Sense in Science."

3. Harold W. Lewis, *Technological Risk*, 94.

4. Berman, *Reenchantment of the World*, 296.

5. Ibid., 275.

6. Steve Martin, *Pure Drivel*, 63–64.

7. Lao Tzu, trans. Feng and English, chap. 8.

·Bibliography

Abrams, Michael. "Eyes in the Back of Your Mouth." *Wired Magazine*, December 2002. www.wired.com/wired/archive/10.12/start.html?pg=9.

Association of Vision Educators. www.visioneducators.org/index.html.

Bache, Christopher M. *Dark Night, Early Dawn: Steps to a Deep Ecology of Mind.* Albany: State University of New York Press, 2000.

Bates, William H. *The Cure of Imperfect Sight by Treatment Without Glasses.* New York: Central Fixation Publishing, 1920. Reprint, Pomeroy, Wash.: Health Research Books, n.d.

———. "A Lesson from the Greeks." *Better Eyesight,* June 1920.

———. "Blindness: Its Causes and Cures." *Better Eyesight,* March 1921.

———. "Common Sense." *Better Eyesight,* June 1923.

———. "Routine Treatment." *Better Eyesight,* December 1927.

———. "Shifting." *Better Eyesight,* December 1925.

———. "Tension." *Better Eyesight,* November 1927.

———. "The Optical Swing." *Better Eyesight,* May 1922.

———. "The Prevention of Myopia: Methods That Failed." *Better Eyesight,* August 1919.

———. "The Vice of Concentration." *Better Eyesight,* July 1921.

———, ed. "A School Teacher's Report, June 12, 1927." *Better Eyesight,* August 1927.

Bates Association for Vision Education (BAVE). www.seeing.org/bave2/bave.htm.

Benjamin, Harry. *Better Sight Without Glasses or Contact Lenses,* 6th ed. London: Thorsons, 1992.

Benson, Herbert. *The Relaxation Response.* New York: Morrow, 1975.

Berenyi, Valerie. "Healthy Rhythms in Drumming." *Star Phoenix* (Saskatoon, SK), August 2, 2003, sec. E3.

Beresford, Stephen M., David W. Muris, Merrill J. Allen, and Francis A. Young. *Improve Your Vision Without Glasses or Contact Lenses.* New York: Simon and Schuster, 1996.

Berman, Morris. *The Reenchantment of the World.* Ithaca, N.Y: Cornell University Press, 1981.

Bernstein, Albert J. *Dinosaur Brains: Dealing with All Those Impossible People at Work.* New York: Wiley, 1989.

Bernstein, Nicholas. *The Co-ordination and Regulation of Movement.* Oxford, 1967. Quoted in Jonathan Cole, *Pride and a Daily Marathon.* Cambridge, Mass.: MIT Press, 1995.

Bittman, Barry. "Deep Within: Drumming as a Healing Strategy." www. mind-body.org/bittman%20deep%20within.htm

Bolles, Mary L. "Learning Abilities' Dramatic Response to Light, Sound, and Motion." In *Light Years Ahead: The Illustrated Guide to Full Spectrum and Colored Light in Mindbody Healing.* Edited by Brian J. Breiling and Bethany ArgIsle. Berkeley, Calif.: Celestial Arts, 1996.

Booth, Jenny. "Concern over Laser Eye Surgery Risks." *News.telegraph,* April 5, 2003. http://portal.telegraph.co.uk/news/main.jhtml?xml-/news/2003/05/ 04/ neye04.xml.

Bowan, Merrill D. "Integrating Vision with the Other Senses." *Neurodevelopmental Optometry,* draft August 8, 1999. www.nb.net/~sparrow/integrate.html.

———. "Stress and the Eye: New Speculations on Refractive Error." *Journal of Behavioral Optometry* 7, no. 5 (1996): 115–22. www.nb.net/~sparrow/ stressandeye.html.

———. "Toward a Unified Theory of Ametropia: Refractive Error as a Lesion." Original title: "Preventing Refractive Error: What's a Doctor to DO?" Available from The Optometric Extension Program as Tape #WK-4 from the 3rd International Congress of Behavioral Optometry. *Perfect Vision Resources.* www.perfectvisionresources.com/news/vision-medical-p-672.htm.

Brofman, Martin. *Improve Your Vision: Your Inner Guide to Clearer Vision.* Forres, Scotland: Findhorn Press, 2004.

Bronowski, Jacob. *The Ascent of Man.* Boston/Toronto: Little, Brown and Company, 1973.

Brown, Otis. "A History of the Origin of the Box-Camera Theory of the Eye: A Question Concerning The Nature of Proof." www.geocities.com/otis brown17268/proveit.txt.

Brumer, Maurice. "Eyestrain: Its Causes, Consequences and Treatment." Australian and New Zealand Association for the Advancement of Science (ANZAAS) Congress, Auckland, New Zealand, 1979. Online at www .myopia.org/brumerpaper.htm.

Calvert, James B. "The Mystery of the Senses." *Brain & Mind: Electronic Magazine on Neuroscience,* December 2002–April 2003. www.cerebro mente.org.br/n16/mente/senses1.html.

Canadian National Institute for the Blind. "CNIB Client Statistics 2002." www .cnib.ca/eng/publications/pamphlets/stats/CNIB_Client_Stats_02_Eng.pdf.

Centers for Disease Control and Prevention (CDC). "*Fusarium* Keratitis— Multiple States, 2006." MMWR Dispatch, April 10, 2006. www.cdc.gov/ mmwr/preview/mmwrhtml/mm55d410a1.htm.

———. "Update: *Fusarium* Keratitis—United States, 2005–2006." MMWR Dispatch, May 19, 2006. www.cdc.gov/mmwr/preview/mmwrhtml/mm55d 519a1.htm.

Chen, Ellen M. *The Tao Te Ching: A New Translation with Commentary.* St. Paul, Minn.: Paragon House, 1989.

Cleary, Thomas. *The Essential Tao: An Initiation into the Heart of Taoism Through the Authentic Tao Te Ching and the Inner Teachings of Chuang-tzu.* San Francisco: Harper Collins, 1991.

Cole, Jonathan. *Pride and a Daily Marathon.* Cambridge: MIT Press, 1995.

Colebrook, Michael. "Emergence." *GreenSpirit.* www.greenspirit.org.uk/resources/ Emergence.htm.

Cousins, Norman. *Anatomy of an Illness as Perceived by the Patient: Reflections on Healing and Regeneration.* New York: Norton, 1979. Reprint, New York: Bantam Books, 1991.

Davies, Clair. *The Trigger Point Therapy Workbook.* Oakland, Calif.: New Harbinger Publications, 2001.

Delwiche, Aaron. "Propaganda: Common Techniques." www.propaganda critic.com.

Dossey, Larry. "Foreword." In Carlyle Hirshberg and Marc Ian Barasch. *Remarkable Recovery: What Extraordinary Healings Tell Us About Getting Well and Staying Well.* New York: Riverhead Books, 1995.

Druker, Samuel. *Optical Journal,* March 15, 1946. Quoted by Alex Eulenberg on International Society for the Enhancement of Eyesight Web site. www.i-see.org/against_glasses.html.

Dubin, Robert. "Post Traumatic Stress Syndrome: Something Can Be Done with Light." In *Light Years Ahead: The Illustrated Guide to Full Spectrum and Colored Light in Mindbody Healing.* Edited by Brian J. Breiling and Bethany ArgIsle. Berkeley, Calif.: Celestial Arts, 1996.

Eisenberg, David M., Roger B. Davis, Susan L. Ettner, et al. "Trends in Alternative Medicine Use in the United States, 1990–1997: Results of a Follow-Up National Survey." *Journal of the American Medical Association* 280, no. 18 (November 1998): 1569–75.

Ekman, Paul. *Emotions Revealed: Recognizing Faces and Feelings to Improve Communication and Emotional Life.* New York: Times Books, 2003.

Feynman, Richard P. "Appendix F: Personal Observations on the Reliability of the Shuttle." In *Report of the Presidential Commission on the Space Shuttle Challenger Accident* (in compliance with Executive Order 12546 of February 3, 1986). Vol. 2. Kennedy Space Center: Science, Technology and Engineering. http://science.ksc.nasa.gov/shuttle/missions/51-l/docs/rogers-commission/table-of-contents.html.

Finando, Donna. *Trigger Point Self-Care Manual.* Rochester, Vt.: Healing Arts Press, 2005.

———. *Trigger Point Therapy For Myofascial Pain.* Rochester, Vt.: Healing Arts Press, 2005.

Francis, W. Nelson. "The English Language and Its History." In *Webster's New Collegiate Dictionary.* Toronto: Thomas Allen and Sons, 1976.

Frost, Robert. "Two Tramps in Mud Time." In *A Further Range,* 1936. Online at American Poems. www.americanpoems.com/poets/robertfrost/772.

Givens, David B. "Eye Blink." Center for Nonverbal Studies (CNS). http://members.aol.com/nonverbal2/eyeblink.htm.

Goethe, Johann Wolfgang von. *Goethes Werke, Hamburger Ausgabe*. Vol. 13, 323. Quoted in Arthur Zajonc, *Catching the Light: The Entwined History of Light and Mind*. New York: Bantam Books, 1993.

Goodrich, Janet. *Natural Vision Improvement*. Berkeley: Celestial Arts, 1986.

Gottlieb, Raymond L. "Neuropsychology of Myopia." *Journal of Optometric Vision Development* 13, no.1 (1982): 3–27.

Gregory, Richard Langton, and Jean G. Wallace. *Recovery from Early Blindness: A Case Study*. Reproduced in March 2001 from Experimental Psychology Society Monograph No. 2, 1963, Cambridge: Heffers. Originally published as *Concepts and Mechanisms of Perception*. London: Duckworth, 1974, 65–129.

Grunwald, Peter. "Peter Grunwald—Profile." Grunwald EyeBody Method. www.eyebody.com/index.cfm?menuID=55.

Heggie, Jack. *Total Body Vision: Lessons to Improve the Quality of Your Vision*. Six audiocassettes and booklet. Lyons, Colo.: Genesis II Publishing, 2001.

Hirshberg, Caryle, and Marc Ian Barasch. *Remarkable Recovery: What Extraordinary Healings Tell Us About Getting Well and Staying Well*. New York: Riverhead Books, 1995.

Huxley, Aldous. *The Art of Seeing*. New York: Harper and Row, 1942. Reprint, with a foreword by Laura Huxley. Berkeley, Calif.: Creative Arts Book Company, 1982.

Illich, Ivan. *Limits to Medicine: Medical Nemesis, the Expropriation of Health*. Enlarged edition. London: Marion Boyars, 1995.

James, William. "Attention." Chap. 11 in *Talks to Teachers on Psychology and to Students on Some of Life's Ideals*. Emory University. www.des.emory.edu/mfp/james.html#talks.

———. *The Principles of Psychology*. Emory University. www.des.emory.edu/mfp/james.html#principles.

Kandinsky, Wassily. *Concerning the Spiritual in Art*. Project Gutenberg EBook, 2004. www.gutenberg.org/dirs/etext04/cnspr10.txt.

Kaplan, Robert-Michael. *The Power Behind Your Eyes: Improving Your Eyesight with Integrated Vision Therapy*. Rochester, Vt.: Healing Arts Press, 1995.

Kaplan, Roberto. *Conscious Seeing: Transforming Your Life Through Your Eyes*. Hillsboro, Ore.: Beyond Words Publishing, 2003.

———. *Seeing Without Glasses: A Step-by-Step Approach to Improving Eyesight Naturally.* 3rd ed. Hillsboro, Ore.: Beyond Words Publishing, 2003.

Kavner, Richard S., and Loraine Dusky. *Total Vision.* New York: Kavner Publishing, 1978.

Keepin, Will. "Lifework of David Bohm: River of Truth." Originally published in *ReVision* 16, no. 1 (summer 1993): 32–46. www.vision.net.au/~apaterson/science/david_bohm.htm.

Kennebeck, Joseph J. *Why Eyeglasses Are Harmful for Children and Young People.* New York: Vantage Press, 1969.

Kiesling, David. "About the Webmaster." Imagination Blindness: The Bates Method of Vision Improvement. www.iblindness.org/aboutme.html.

———. "Signs of Progress." Imagination Blindness: The Bates Method of Vision Improvement. www.iblindness.org/intro/progress.html.

Klemons, Ira. "Chest Pain and Headaches." www.headandfacialpain.com/pain.html.

Lakatos, Imre. "Science and Pseudoscience." Transcript of June 30, 1973, Programme 11 of The Open University Arts Course A303, "Problems of Philosophy." London School of Economics and Political Science. www.lse.ac.uk/collections/lakatos//scienceAndPseudoscienceTranscript.htm.

Langer, Ellen J. *Mindfulness.* Cambridge, Mass.: Perseus Books, 1989.

Lao Tzu. *Tao Te Ching.* In *Tao Te Ching: A New English Version, with Foreword and Notes,* translated by Stephen Mitchell. New York: Harper Collins, 1988.

———. *Tao Te Ching.* In *The Tao Te Ching: A New Translation with Commentary,* translated by Ellen M. Chen. St. Paul, Minn.: Paragon House, 1989.

———. *Tao Te Ching.* In *The Essential Tao: An Initiation into the Heart of Taoism Through the Authentic Tao Te Ching and the Inner Teachings of Chuang-tzu,* translated by Thomas Cleary. San Francisco: Harper Collins, 1991.

———. *Tao Te Ching.* Translated by Gia-fu Feng and Jane English. 25th Anniversary ed. New York: Vintage Books, 1997.

Levinson, Harold N. *Phobia Free.* With Stephen Carter. New York: M. Evans and Company, 1986.

Leviton, Richard. *Seven Steps to Better Vision.* Brookline, Mass.: East West/Natural Health Books, 1992.

Lewin, Roger. "Is Your Brain Really Necessary?" *Science* 210 (new series), no. 4475 (December 12, 1980): 1232–34.

Lewis, Harold W. *Technological Risk.* New York: W. W. Norton, 1990.

Lewis, Hunter. *A Question of Values: Six Ways We Make the Personal Choices That Shape Our Lives.* New York: Harper and Row, 1990.

Liberman, Jacob. *Light: Medicine of the Future.* Rochester, Vt.: Bear and Company, 1991.

———. *Take Off Your Glasses and See.* New York: Three Rivers Press, 1995.

Lierman, Emily C. "Individual Treatment." *Better Eyesight,* February 1928.

———. "Stories from the Clinic, 11: A Case of Cataract." *Better Eyesight,* January 1921.

Lightle, Jane, ed. "Cancer: Can You Lower Your Risk?" *Wellness Matters.* North Vancouver, BC: Seajay Communications Ltd., Fall 2003, 8.

Link, Ron. "Complications." Surgical Eyes. www.surgicaleyes.org/complications.htm.

———. "Why We're Here." Surgical Eyes. www.surgicaleyes.org/WhyHere .htm.

Lowen, Alexander. *The Language of the Body.* New York: Grune and Stratton, 1958. Quoted in Raymond L. Gottlieb, "Neuropsychology of Myopia," *Journal of Optometric Vision Development* 13, no. 1 (1982): 3–27.

MacDonald, Glynn. *The Complete Illustrated Guide to the Alexander Technique.* Boston: Element Books, 1998.

MacFarlane, Alan, and Gerry Martin. *Glass: A World History.* Chicago: University of Chicago Press, 2002.

———. "Preliminary Drafts on Glass: Chapter 16." www.alanmacfarlane.com/ glass/texts.html.

Martin, Nicolas S. "Promoting Accountability for Medical Professionals and Institutions." American Iatrogenic Association. www.iatrogenic.org.

Martin, Steve. *Pure Drivel.* New York: Hyperion, 1998.

McCaffey, Barbara. "Burning, Stinging, Gritty Eyes?" Canadian Diabetes Care Guide. www.diabetescareguide.com/articles/dryeye.htm.

Mew, John. "Common Sense in Science." Natural Growth Guidance: The Alternative to Straightening Teeth with Extractions, and Surgery. www.orthotropics.com/patients_parents/commonsense.html.

Mihoces, Gary. "You've Got to See 130-mph Serve to Return It." *USA Today,*

February 25, 2003. www.usatoday.com/sports/2003-02-24-ten-hardest-tennis-return_x.htm.

Miller, Dick. *Triumphant Journey: The Saga of Bobby Jones and the Grand Slam of Golf.* New York: Holt, Reinhart and Winston, 1980. Reprint, Grass Valley, Calif.: The Booklegger, 1991.

Mills, Stephanie, ed. *Turning Away from Technology: A New Vision for the 21st Century.* San Francisco: Sierra Club Books, 1997.

Mitchell, Stephen. *Tao Te Ching: A New English Version.* New York: Harper Collins, 1988.

Mumford, Lewis. *The Pentagon of Power.* Vol. 2, *The Myth of the Machine.* New York: Harcourt Brace Jovanovich, 1970.

National Academies' Institute of Medicine. *To Err Is Human: Building a Safer Health System (2000).* Washington, D.C.: National Academies Press, 2000, 26–27.

National Institute on Deafness and Other Communication Disorders, National Institutes of Health. "Ménière's Disease." www.nidcd.nih.gov/health/balance/meniere.asp.

National Mental Health Institute, "Depression Can Break Your Heart: A brief overview of the relationship between depression and heart disease." 2001. www.nimh.nih.gov/publicat/heartbreak.cfm.

———. "Reliving Trauma: Post-Traumatic Stress Disorder: A brief overview of the symptoms, treatments, and research findings." 2001. www.nimh.nih.gov/publicat/reliving.cfm.

———. "The Numbers Count: Mental Disorders in America: A summary of statistics describing the prevalence of mental disorders in America." 2006 (rev). www.nimh.nih.gov/publicat/numbers.cfm#readNow.

National Research Council, Committee on Vision. *Myopia: Prevalence and Progression.* Washington, D.C.: National Academy Press, 1989.

Nearing, Helen, and Scott Nearing. *The Good Life: Helen and Scott Nearing's Sixty Years of Self-Sufficient Living.* Reprint (2 vols. in 1, *Living the Good Life,* 1970, and *Continuing the Good Life,* 1979). New York: Schocken Books, 1989.

Null, Gary, and Debora Rasio. "Iatrogenic Illness: The Downside of Modern Medicine." 2000. http://gnhealth.com/scripts/prodView.asp?idproduct =1050.

Orfield, Antonia. "Seeing Space: Undergoing Brain Re-Programming to Reduce

Myopia." *Journal of Behavioral Optometry* 5, no. 5 (1994). Optometrists Network. www.optometrists.org/Boston/articles.html.

Orlock, Carol. *Know Your Body Clock.* New York: Carol Publishing Group, 1995.

Pearce, Joseph Chilton. *Evolution's End: Claiming the Potential of Our Intelligence.* San Francisco: Harper San Francisco, 1993.

Peat, F. David. "Blackfoot Physics and European Minds." www.fdavidpeat .com/bibliography/essays/black.htm.

———. "Creativity and Education." www.fdavidpeat.com/bibliography/essays/ dempsey.htm.

Polanyi, Michael. *Personal Knowledge.* Chicago: University of Chicago Press, 1962, 101. Quoted in Morris Berman, *The Reenchantment of the World.* Ithaca, N.Y.: Cornell University Press, 1981.

Preidt, Robert. "Eye-Opening British Study Under Way: Photoreceptors in Our Eyes Influence Our Internal Body Clocks." *HealthScout,* December 2, 2000. www.oobdoo.net/online/inter-change.subportal.com/Health/inter-change .subportal.com/health/Health_Biz/Devices_Technologies/Biotechnology/ 103359.html.

Prudden, Bonnie. *Pain Erasure: The Bonnie Prudden Way.* New York: Ballantine Books, 1982.

Pulos, Lee, and Gary Richman. *Miracles and Other Realities.* San Francisco: Omega Press, 1990.

Quackenbush, Thomas R. *Relearning to See.* Berkeley: North Atlantic Books, 1997.

———, ed. *Better Eyesight: The Complete Magazines of William H. Bates.* Berkeley: North Atlantic Books, 2001.

Rach2 [username]. "Lonely and Frustrated." Eye-Openers, Personal Post-Op Stories, posted January 30, 2003. Vision Surgery Rehab Network. www .surgicaleyes.infopop.cc/groupee/forums/a/tpc/f/6541031211/m/3496066494.

Raphaelson, Jacob. *Spectacle Hobby: A Story with a Purpose.* Cincinnati: Research Foundation for Prevention of Myopia, 1961. Quoted at International Society for the Enhancement of Eyesight. www.i-see.org/ against_glasses.html.

Ribe, Neil, and Friedrich Steinle. "Exploratory Experimentation: Goethe, Land,

and Color Theory." PhysicsToday.org, July 2002. www.physicstoday.org/
vol-55/iss-7/p43.html.

Robbins, Anthony. *Unlimited Power.* New York: Fawcett Columbine, 1987.

Rooney, Andy. "Saddam's Capture: Extra, Extra!" *60 Minutes,* CBS News,
December 14, 2003. www.cbsnews.com/stories/2003/12/14/60minutes/
rooney/main588520.shtml.

Sahlins, Marshall. "The Original Affluent Society." In *Stone Age Economics.* New
York: Aldine, 1972, 1–39. www.primitivism.com/original-affluent.htm.

Savan, Beth. *Science Under Siege: The Myth of Objectivity in Scientific Research.*
Toronto: CBC Enterprises, 1988.

Schneider, Meir, and Maureen Larkin. *The Handbook of Self-Healing.* With
Dror Schneider. New York: Penguin Putnam, 1994.

Schneider, Meir. *Self-Healing: My Life and Vision.* New York: Arkana, Penguin
Group, 1989.

Selye, Hans. *Stress Without Distress.* New York: New American Library, 1975.

———. *The Stress of Life,* rev. ed. New York: McGraw-Hill, 1976.

Shelton, Herbert M. *Natural Hygiene: The Pristine Way of Life.* 2d ed. Tampa,
Fla.: American Natural Hygiene Society, 1994.

Smith, Huston. *The World's Religions: Our Great Wisdom Traditions.* New
York: Harper Collins, 1991.

Steiner, Rudolf. *How to Know the Higher Worlds: A Modern Path of Initiation.*
Translated by Christopher Bamford. Herndon, Va.: Anthroposophic Press,
1994.

———. *Polarities in Health, Illness and Therapy.* Lecture, Pennmenmawr, N.
Wales, August 28, 1923. Spring Valley, NY: Mercury Press, 1987. Rudolf
Steiner Archive. http://wn.rsarchive.org/Lectures/Polart_index.html.

———. *Theosophy: An Introduction to the Spiritual Processes in Human Life
and in the Cosmos.* Translated by Catherine E. Creeger. Herndon, Va.:
Anthroposophic Press, 1994. First English edition published 1910 by Kegan
Paul, London and Rand McNally, Chicago.

Stevenson, Ian. "Some of My Journeys in Medicine." The 1989 Flora Levy Lecture
in the Humanities, University of Southwestern Louisiana, Lafayette, La. www.
healthsystem.virginia.edu/internet/personalitystudies/some-of-my-journeys-
in-medicine.pdf.

Suzuki, David. "An Erratic Journey Through Science and Society." Chap. 8 in *Beyond the Ivory Tower: Public Intellectuals, Academia and the Media.* Edited by Saleem Ali and Robert Barsky. Massachusetts Institute of Technology. www.mit.edu/~saleem/ivory/ch8.htm.

Twain, Mark. "Blind Tom." Correspondence with the San Francisco *Alta California,* August 1, 1869. www.twainquotes.com/18690801.html.

U.K. Department of Social Security, Corporate Medical Group. *Stress Related Illness: A Report for DSS Policy Group.* Part 1, February 1998. Department for Work and Pensions. www.dwp.gov.uk/medical/sreport1.pdf.

———. *Stress Related Illness: A Report for DSS Policy Group.* Part 2, February 1998. Department for Work and Pensions. www.dwp.gov.uk/medical/sreport2.pdf.

Upledger, John E. *Your Inner Physician and You: CranioSacral Therapy and SomatoEmotional Release.* Berkeley, Calif.: North Atlantic Books; Palm Beach Gardens, Fla.: UI Enterprises, 1997.

Vision Council of America. "Sales, Purchase Intent Rise during the First Quarter." www.visionsite.org/s_vision/doc.asp?CID=270&DID=1959.

von Senden, M. *Space and Sight: The Perception of Space and Shape in the Congenitally Blind Before and After Operation.* Translated by Peter Heath. Glencoe, Ill.: The Free Press, 1960, 160. Quoted in Arthur Zajonc, *Catching the Light: The Entwined History of Light and Mind.* New York: Bantam Books, 1993, 6.

WrongDiagnosis.com. "Symptom: Blurred Vision." www.wrongdiagnosis.com/sym/blurred_vision.htm.

Young, Emma. "Controversial Dyslexia Treatment 'Works.'" NewScientist.com, November 5, 2002. www.newscientist.com/news/news.jsp?id=ns99993012.

Zajonc, Arthur. *Catching the Light: The Entwined History of Light and Mind.* New York: Bantam Books, 1993.

Index

BOOKS OF RELATED INTEREST

Light: Medicine of the Future
How We Can Use It to Heal Ourselves NOW
by Jacob Liberman, O.D., Ph.D.

The Power Behind Your Eyes
Improving Your Eyesight with Integrated Vision Therapy
by Robert-Michael Kaplan, O.D.

How to Improve Your Child's Eyesight Naturally
A Thoughtful Parent's Guide
by Janet Goodrich, Ph.D.

Chi Self-Massage
The Taoist Way of Rejuvenation
by Mantak Chia

Tao of No Stress
Three Simple Paths
by Stuart Alve Olson

The Tao of Detox
The Secrets of Yang-Sheng Dao
by Daniel Reid

The Detox Mono Diet
The Miracle Grape Cure and Other Cleansing Diets
by Christopher Vasey, N.D.

Facial Reflexology
A Self-Care Manual
by Marie-France Muller, M.D., N.D., Ph.D.

Inner Traditions • Bear & Company
P.O. Box 388
Rochester, VT 05767
1-800-246-8648
www.InnerTraditions.com

Or contact your local bookseller